David Rieff is a contributing writer to *The New York Times Magazine*. He is the author of seven previous books, including the acclaimed *At the Point of a Gun: Democratic Dreams and Armed Intervention*, *A Bed for the Night: Humanitarianism in Crisis* and *Slaughterhouse Bosnia and the Failure of the West*. He lives in New York City.

'Susan Sontag was fiercely, exuberantly alive, and uncompromising in her life no less than her work. David Rieff's fine, tender, and unflinching portrait of her final illness brings home her absolute determination to survive to the last – to survive against the odds and live creatively despite a devastating disease and an unproven cancer treatment. At once a report from the frontlines of experimental oncology and a moving, absorbing personal account of his mother's last illness, *Swimming in the Sea of Death* is a courageous and darkly beautiful book' Oliver Sacks

'This is a sad and sombre book, but it's leavened with wise quotations. And, like Joan Didion's *The Year of Magical Thinking*, its story of an embattled death-refusenik is the more affecting because it sheds no tears' Blake Morrison, *Guardian*

ALSO BY DAVID RIEFF

SWIMMING IN A SEA OF DEATH

A Son's Memoir

DAVID RIEFF

GRANTA

Granta Publications, 12 Addison Avenue, London W11 4QR

First published in Great Britain by Granta Books, 2008
First published in the US in 2008 by Simon & Schuster, Inc.
This paperback edition first published by Granta Books, 2009

Excerpt from "Aubade" from *Collected Poems* by Philip Larkin.
Copyright © 1988, 2003 by the Estate of Philip Larkin. Reprinted by
permission of Faber & Faber. Excerpt from *Sloan-Kettering: Poems* by
Abba Kovner, translated by Eddie Levenston. Copyright © 2002 by the
Estate of Abba Kovner. Foreword copyright © 2002 by Leon
Wieseltier. Reprinted by permission of Schocken Books, a division of
Random House, Inc. Excerpt from "When in my White Room at the
Charité" from *Bertolt Brecht: Poems 1913–1956* by Bertolt Brecht,
edited by John Willett and Ralph Manheim, with the co-operation of
Erich Fried. Routledge 1997. Reprinted by permission of the Taylor &
Francis Group. Excerpt from *The Complete Poetry: A Bilingual
Edition* by César Vallejo, edited and translated by Clayton Eshleman.
With a Foreword by Mario Vargas Llosa, an Introduction by Efraín
Kristal, and a Chronology by Stephen M. Hart. Copyright © 2007 by
The Regents of the University of California. Reprinted by permission of
the University of California Press.

A CIP catalogue record for this book
is available from the British Library.

1 3 5 7 9 10 8 6 4 2

ISBN 978 1 84708 075 2

Printed in the UK by CPI Bookmarque, Croydon, CR0 4TD

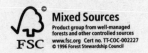

Mixed Sources
Product group from well-managed
forests and other controlled sources
www.fsc.org Cert no. TT-COC-002227
© 1996 Forest Stewardship Council

FSC

For Miranda

Because I know that time is always time

And place is always and only place

And what is actual is actual only for one time

And only for one place

I rejoice that things are as they are and

I renounce the blessèd face.

T. S. ELIOT
Ash Wednesday, 1930

SWIMMING IN
A SEA OF DEATH

I

NOTHING could have been further from my mind. I thought that I was returning to my home in New York at the end of a long trip abroad. Instead, I was at the beginning of the journey that would end with my mother's death.

To be specific, it was the afternoon of March 28, 2004, a Sunday, and I was in Heathrow Airport in London on my way back from the Middle East. After almost a month moving back and forth between East Jerusalem and the West Bank (I had been writing a magazine story about the Palestinians in the last period of Arafat's rule), I was relieved to be going home, and now I was halfway there. Other than that, though, my mind was pretty much a blank. The trip had been frustrating and I had only partly succeeded in getting what I needed. I knew that writing up the story was bound to be difficult. But I was tired, and both a little burnt out and a little hung over, and I was not yet ready to try to turn my reporting into writing. That could wait until I got home, and so instead, in the United Airlines lounge, I began making phone calls—reconnecting with home as has always been my habit once I am through reporting a story. That was when my mother, Susan Sontag, told me that there was a chance that she was ill again.

My mother was clearly doing her best to be cheerful. "There *may* be something wrong," she finally told me after I had gone on at far too great length about what the West Bank had been like. While I had been away, she said, she had gone in for her twice-yearly scans and blood tests—the regular routine that she had been following since her surgery and subsequent chemotherapy for the uterine sarcoma she had been diagnosed with six years earlier. "One of the blood tests they've just run doesn't seem so good," she said, adding that she had already had some further tests done, and asking me if I

would come with her the following day to see a specialist who had been recommended to her and who had
done some follow-up tests a couple of days earlier. He
would have the conclusive results then. "It's probably
nothing," she said, and reminded me of the long list of
false alarms that had come up in the aftermath of both
her sarcoma and the radical mastectomy she had under-
gone after being diagnosed with advanced breast cancer in 1975.

She repeated that it was probably nothing. Inanely,
I repeated it, too. We were agreed on that, we told each
other. In theory, at least, it wasn't completely irrational
for us both to say this. None of those false alarms had
ever amounted to anything, had they? There had been
that time when a scan had revealed something in her
left kidney. It, too, had looked like cancer, but in the
end it had turned out that my mother simply had an
oddly shaped kidney. Then there had been the time
when my mother's doctors worried that a sudden onset
of severe stomach cramps might mean colon cancer.
Those fears, too, had proved groundless. And having
lived, as everyone who has had cancer does, with this

sword of Damocles of a recurrence over her head since she contracted her first cancer in her early forties, my mother had learned the hard way to be calm when she received such news, or, at least, to act calmly. This, too, would be a false alarm, we each said again. Hadn't we been over this ground before? But our words were like shallow breaths and our composure built of numbness rather than calm. I'm ashamed to say that I was relieved when we rang off.

Afterward, I tried not to think of anything, staring out at the runways of Heathrow, watching the planes land and take off, until I heard the boarding call for my own flight. Once on the plane, I got drunk, but then I always do. After we landed, I went home. When I arrived, I called my mother's apartment, but it was a friend of hers who answered and she told me that my mother was sleeping. I said I was going to do the same. And did. The alternative was screaming with the pain of believing that this time there might be no reprieve. I can't even imagine what it must have been like for her.

The following morning, I went to collect my mother at her apartment. Far from being rested, it was immediately obvious to me that she had not slept. Thinking back, I remember her frantic cheeriness, and my only partly successful efforts to mimic it. I say "partly successful" because, although I was able to remain calm, there already seemed to be the tiniest pause between my saying something and my hearing myself say it. Thinking back, I wish I'd hugged her close or held her hand. But neither of us had ever been physically demonstrative with the other, and while much has been said and written about how people transcend their pettier sides in crises, in my experience, at least, what actually happens is that more often we reveal what lies beneath the waterline of what we essentially are. What my mother and I shared were words and yet now they felt all but valueless—like Confederate dollars or Soviet roubles. I do not remember my own fear, but I remember vividly imagining hers. And yet she kept on talking about the Middle East, and, unable to say anything that mattered, let alone touch her, I kept on telling stories about Yasir Arafat and his compound in Ramallah—as if that mattered anymore. This conversation went on until we arrived at the specialist's office—or, more precisely, the leukemia specialist's office.

Dr. A.—feeling about him as I do, I prefer not to name him—was a large man with an outsized (and to me overbearing) manner to fit his girth. Or so it seemed to me. Perhaps had he had better news to convey, or even a better manner in delivering bad news, I might have retained another image of him—Friar Tuck, perhaps, or some jolly Dickens character. And in fairness to him, by then I was both almost catatonic with dread and increasingly disoriented psychically. Everything had shifted, I felt, and I could no longer tell the solid from the flimsy. It was all I could do to shake Dr. A.'s hand, smile mechanically at some remark he made about traveling journalists, and sit down next to my mother. I do remember looking intently at him across his wide, cluttered desk as he delivered the bad news. For it wasn't "nothing." To the contrary, it was, unthinkably, everything. Dr. A. was quite clear. From the tests that he had done the previous Friday—blood workups and a bone marrow biopsy—he was in absolutely no doubt that my mother had myelodysplastic syndrome.

My mother and I both stared at him blankly. The word meant nothing to either of us. Our befuddlement, his frustration. MDS, he explained, slowly and deliberately, as if he had a family of village idiots sitting in front of him, was a particularly lethal form of blood cancer.

"Say something," I thought to myself. My head was throbbing. Trying to mimic Dr. A.'s tone, I managed to ask him if he was absolutely certain? Didn't many cancers have similar presentations? I asked, seeking asylum in medical jargon much as he seemed to be taking refuge in acronyms and pedagogy. Was there any room for doubt, any chance of there being just *something* wrong, and of that "something" turning out to be something less lethal? Dr. A. shook his head emphatically. The blood tests and, above all, the bone marrow biopsy, he said, were completely unambiguous. He then went on to explain what MDS was. I listened without really hearing, listened in a daze as these unfamiliar words and terms cascaded out of him, leaving him successfully enough but not quite reaching me. MDS was marked by "refractory anemia," he said. The stem cells that my mother's bone marrow was producing were no longer developing into mature blood cells but instead were remaining "blasts"—immature blood cells that could not function normally.

I did not take any of this in at the time, except, of course, that the news was terrible. Given his experience, I have to assume that Dr. A. knew that his words were unlikely to be understood at the first go-around. Like so many doctors, he spoke to us as if we were children but without the care that a sensible adult takes in choosing what words to use with a child. Instead, he proceeded as if in a lecture hall. Neither my mother nor I interrupted him.

After he had finished, though, my mother asked Dr. A. what treatments were being used for MDS, and what were the chances of remission from the disease? Again, he made no effort to prepare her for what he was about to say or to put it in a fashion that expressed any particular sympathy for her or any horror at my mother's situation. If all doctors behaved in this way, I could forgive him. But all doctors do not behave this way, as, thankfully, my mother would subsequently discover.

Dr. A. warmed to his theme. For all intents and purposes, he replied, the answer was that there were no treatments that did that much good, or at least none that could induce a long-term remission, let alone a cure. Of course, there were a number of palliative drugs, drugs to improve the patient's "quality of life." This expression—call it medical cliché, euphemism, or medical term of art—was one that doctors and nurses would repeat constantly throughout my mother's illness. Dr. A. went on to say that there was one drug called 5-azacitidine that could often induce a temporary remission. But it usually was effective for no more than six months at the most. Apart from "5-aza," though, really the only way to survive with MDS for very long was to get a bone marrow transplant. But that, Dr. A. said, wasn't a very promising avenue for a woman of seventy-one like my mother. Indeed, Dr. A.'s recommendation was that my mother do nothing until the MDS "converted"—the use of the word was one with which I was totally unfamiliar but that I would come to know and dread—into "full-blown" AML, acute myeloid leukemia.

Why this was so was not immediately clear to me. To the contrary, waiting seemed suicidal since AML, it appeared, was far worse even than MDS (and how quickly these acronyms began to implant themselves in one's consciousness). In AML, the stem cells developed into abnormal white and red blood cells and platelets. The more of these so-called leukemia cells or blasts there were, the less room there could be for healthy blood cells and platelets. What this meant was that once the number of leukemia cells in the blood and bone marrow reached a certain threshold, the body could no longer maintain its functions. Dr. A. did not articulate the obvious corollary, which was that after that, one died. He did not need to. That much my mother and I *had* understood.

My mother still had on the rigid smile she had worn as I told her Middle East stories on the drive from her apartment up to Dr. A.'s office. But as Dr. A. kept speaking I had the strongest illusion that I actually could hear it cracking like an eggshell. But I realized that I was looking away from her, away from Dr. A., at the birthday greetings celebrating his recent fiftieth birthday, at his books, at his family photographs—anywhere, in fact, except at my mother. So I cannot say for sure. I do know that it was some time before she spoke.

"So what you're telling me," she finally said, with a

poignant deliberation that makes me gasp even remembering it, "is that in fact there is nothing to be done." After a pause, she added, "Nothing I can do."

Dr. A. did not answer directly, but his silence was, as the cliché goes, eloquent. A few minutes later, after delivering the requisite invitation for my mother to come back and see him after she had thought through what she wanted to do next—I remember finding that word, "wanted," particularly grotesque—we left. The silence in which we walked to the car was beyond anything I could have imagined or had ever experienced. On the drive downtown, she stared out the window. Then, after five minutes or so, she turned away from the window and back toward me.

"Wow," she said. "Wow."

IT CANNOT be true statistically that the worst things that happen to you in life always happen when you least expect them. But when terrible things do happen, that is what one almost always feels. Perhaps this is just as well. After all, the alternative to *not* expecting the worst would be all but unbearable. There is a play by Elias Canetti whose premise is that the characters all go about their business wearing lockets around their necks that state the year in which they will die. And the play's premise is its point: to live with such knowledge would turn the experience of living into little more than an antechamber to extinction.

I suppose Canetti comes into my mind not only because my mother loved his work, and even once wrote an essay about him that I found to be as much disguised autobiography as it was one writer describing another's work, but because what she cherished most about it, and even more than the work about Canetti the man, I think, was his fear of death. More precisely, she shared his complete inability, whether as a young man or in great age, to reconcile himself to the fact of mortality. "I curse death," he wrote, "I cannot help it." You could almost say that his argument, like hers, was with the book of Genesis. In one of her early journals— my mother was then a sixteen-year-old student at the University of Chicago—she writes of "not being able to even imagine that one day I will no longer be alive."

Like Canetti, she carried this sentiment, normal to the point of banality in a young person, almost until the moment she died in the Memorial Sloan-Kettering Cancer Center, a little less than three weeks before her seventy-second birthday.

What I am trying to convey is that she died as she had lived: unreconciled to mortality, even after suffering so much pain—and God, what pain she suffered! In spite of all that, my mother stood with Canetti, and with Philip Larkin who, in his great poem "Aubade," wrote of his dread of dying and his disdain for religious consolation and other mental tricks:

> *. . . And specious stuff that says No rational being*
> *Can fear a thing it will not feel, not seeing*
> *That this is what we fear—no sight, no sound,*
> *No touch or taste or smell, nothing to think with,*
> *Nothing to love or link with,*
> *The anaesthetic from which none come round.*

Reading these lines that I have known since I memorized them when I was young—though for me now they no longer conjure up Larkin's bald head and pursed lips but rather my mother's wild black-and-white mane of hair and the intensity of her dark eyes—I want so badly to temporize with her. "Don't love life so much," I want to say, "you always rated it too highly." Or else I want to console her, all the while knowing that she was no more consolable than Larkin was, or than I am for that matter. But I want to try, and, as I imagine it (irrationally), grant her some tiny sliver of acceptance of death, or, if not that, perhaps at least confer upon her some flake of Buddhist indifference to extinction. I want to remind her of a day in the late seventies when a woman with breast cancer came to see her and told her she was not interested in Western medical treatment because it could only offer remission, whereas she was interested in cure. "But we're all in remission," my mother told her. I'd like to remind her she said that. I'd like to make a "case for the defense" *for* mortality.

But if I am being honest with myself, I have to admit that I don't think it would have done any good at all, by which I mean it would not have strengthened, or armed, or consoled her. There was an eighteenth-century French writer who wrote a friend asking "why, hating life as I do, do I fear death so much?" That was Larkin's perspective, too. It was even Canetti's when he wrote, "One should not confuse the craving for life with endorsement of it." But it was not my mother's. She loved living and, if anything, both her appetite for experience and her hopes for what she would accomplish as a writer had only increased as she grew older. If I had to choose one word to describe her way of being in the world it would be "avidity." There was nothing she did not want to see or do or try to know.

In a strange way, she lived her life as if stocking a library, or materializing her longings—many of them unchanged since lonely girlhood. She never said this, but I wonder if her sense of herself was not inextricably bound up in this collecting—the subject of so much of her best writing. In another of her diaries, she writes that she is an eternal student and speculates whether, in the end, that is what she is best at. She wanted to absorb; she did not want to be absorbed—and certainly not to be absorbed into eternity, into nothingness. Why . . . no, how, could she have wanted to close the library down and disperse its holdings to the wind, never to be reconstituted? "Where I am, death is not," Epicurus wrote, "where death is, I am not." But then, as my mother wrote, she could only imagine *being*.

The fancy that I could have consoled her is itself presumptuous. She who could talk about anything could rarely really speak of death directly, though I believe that she thought about it constantly. I remember that when I was very small, and, stricken, was just coming to understand what mortality was—for some odd reason it had been a statue of George Washington that had set me off: the great man "wasn't"—I tried to talk with her about it. I was desperately upset, and if not weeping, then on the verge of doing so, and she did what she could to console me. But even then, I remember noticing through the scrim of my own distress how upset she herself quickly became. And it was not long before I had the dim sense that it was I who should be consoling *her*, not asking for consolation. "There may be some strange, chemical immortality," she told me, and then, voice trailing off, she added, "but too late for either of us, I'm afraid."

I was too young to do anything for her then, of course. But how I would have liked to have been able somehow to console her, after that meeting with Dr. A. and through the months of her illness until her death. But instead, almost until the moment she died, we talked of her survival, of her struggle with cancer, never about her dying. I was not going to raise the subject unless she did. It was her death, not mine. And she did not raise it. To have done so would have been to concede that she might die and what she wanted was survival, not extinction—survival on any terms. To go on living: perhaps that was her way of dying.

IN RETROSPECT, looking at the photographs of my mother taken in the year before she was diagnosed, I think I can discern that she was ill already. There is something about her color, a pastiness, a pallor, and also something in her expression—pained is too weak a word for it, though there is pain in her eyes—that seem to scream out that she is in trouble. But of course I have no idea if in fact her illness was already so evident or whether I am reading all this into the pictures I have of her from this period. The National Cancer Institute's Web page about MDS identifies "having skin that is paler than usual," shortness of breath, fever, tiredness, and easy bruising or bleeding as possible signs of the disease. But then, these are signs of many diseases other than cancer and she did not act as if she were ill. If anything, her always-busy schedule was even more packed than usual, and her energies as prodigious as they had ever been. She traveled, she lectured, she wrote, all the while finding time to pursue her passions for theater, dance, and film. People half her age (and as she got older, she increasingly preferred the company of much younger people) could barely keep up with her, something that gave her enormous pleasure.

Am I supposed to be ironic about what, in retrospect, was to be the last of her Indian summers, perhaps quoting the P. G. Wodehouse line about how "unseen, in the background, Fate was quietly slipping the lead into the boxing glove," which of course it was? Or am I to ascribe some special meaning to the intensity of her final years, as if somehow she had a premonition that her time was ending? Or is all of this just that vain, irrational human wish to ascribe meaning when no meaning is really on offer?

What I can say without any sentimental speculation or reading back from the end of the story, while all the while knowing how it finished, is that despite her fear of death, she lived as if she were going to live for a long time more. Characteristically, she spoke of "needing" the time to do all the writing that she still had in her. And more and more frequently, not just on birthdays and other enforced contemplations of mortality, she spoke of wanting to live to be a hundred. In the past, she often told me, she had done too many things she hadn't wanted to do. Now, she said, she was finally going to do the work that really mattered to her. Above all, she was going to write more fiction. She just needed the time to do it. Fate and boxing gloves: perhaps there is nothing ironic about the conceit after all.

I do not know this, but my sense is that she had always lived in the future. During her childhood, which was profoundly unhappy, she fantasized of her future existence as an adult, unshackled from her family from which she felt so removed. And during her intense but finally disordered and impossible marriage to my father, I believe she fantasized of an independent life for herself in New York—a writer's life, not that of the academic she had been. As an essayist, she dreamt of the novels she would write. So, again and again, I look at her life's trajectory and see the future tense elbowing out the present. And yet surely the only way to even remotely come to terms with death is to live in the present. If you get to act three and you are still expecting two acts to come, the prospect of a final exit *is* unbearable. There is no way to reconcile oneself to it. Anyway, that is the way it was for my mother. She would not contemplate extinction until the last month of her life. And even then . . . Instead, throughout most of her illness, she was still interested in compiling lists of restaurants and books, quotations and facts, writing projects and travel schedules, all of which I understood to be her way of fighting to the end for another shard of the future.

Which was her right. I'm sure of that. What I'm far less sure of is whether I did the right thing in going along with and in fact doing what I could to abet her in her refusal to contemplate the prospect that this third time around she would die of her cancer. Looked at from a distance, this is probably just one variant of what you might call "the loved one's dilemma." The questions tumble out, in wakefulness and in dreams. At least, more than two years after her death, they continue to for me: Did I do the right thing? Could I have done more? Or proposed an alternative? Or been more supportive? Or forced the issue of death to the fore? Or concealed it better?

The unanswerable questions of a survivor.

II

My MOTHER had lived almost her entire seventy-one years believing that she was a person who would beat the odds, no matter how steep they seemed. In this, as in so much else in her life, she remained determined, and as consistent in old age as she had been in childhood. Above all, it was that childhood, about which she often described herself as having felt "abandoned and unloved," that remained the touchstone both of resistance and of ambition—two ideas that for her were never entirely separable. "My earliest childhood decision," she wrote in her journal, "By God, they won't get me." What this meant for her, she added, was an "absolute decision not to be done in."

Obviously, she was not alluding to being done in by illness, though she was crippled by asthma as a girl, but rather by her mother, whose coldness and withholding nature (my mother's words, again) so haunted her, or by her jovial, war hero stepfather (her real father died in China when she was four) who, meaning absolutely no harm, nonetheless would tell her constantly—or at least, so she experienced it—that she shouldn't read so much if she ever hoped to find a good husband. My mother herself never doubted that it was this will to survive, ignoring the conventional wisdom, to bounce back, to thrive against all odds, that had given her this paradoxical conviction of being a lucky person—that is, of having a good chance at being the exception in whatever situation she found herself. It had also, she sometimes told me, turned her into the risk-taker that she would become as an adult.

But all this effort that she had put in to shaping herself into the person she had first dreamt of being while still a solitary, asthmatic ten-year-old in southern Arizona would serve her well when, in 1975, she was diagnosed with advanced breast cancer that had spread into seventeen of her lymph nodes. In her essay "AIDS and Its Metaphors," written over ten years after her illness, she would reminisce a little proudly of "confounding my doctors' pessimism." And when she spoke of their pessimism, she was putting it mildly. What I don't think she ever knew, what I never told her in any case, was that William Cahan, at that time her principal doctor at Memorial Sloan-Kettering Cancer Center in New York City, never really expected her to live. That was what he had told me either the first or second time we had a moment alone together after he had admitted her to the hospital.

Those were the days in which it was standard practice for doctors to lie to cancer patients. If they were candid at all, it was usually by opting to deliver all bad news to family members instead of leveling with their patients. Of course, attitudes were changing even then, and some American physicians were beginning to take seriously what at the time seemed like the revolutionary ideas of patient autonomy and informed consent that today are routinely taught—whether effectively or ineffectively is another matter—at American medical schools.

But for the most part in those days, most physicians shared a set of assumptions about how much truth to tell and to whom that had led ninety percent of American oncologists surveyed in 1961 for an article published by the *Journal of the American Medical Association* to admit that they would not tell their patients that they had cancer.

Bill Cahan was still very much of this school. What he thought I, as a family member, was supposed to then do with the death sentence he had pronounced was not something he ever said. And I was at first too stunned, and then too frightened, to ask him to elaborate. I suspect my experience was typical for the time. I remember pacing the corridors of the breast cancer floor at Memorial Hospital wondering what to tell my mother and what not to tell her. To do so seemed like sadism. But not to do so seemed like betrayal. In the end, I did nothing.

Still, even if I chose to remain silent (if "chose" is even the right word), and if Bill Cahan and her other principal doctors were not willing to level with her, my mother certainly knew that the odds were that she would die. Nothing anyone said or didn't say could occlude the fact that her cancer was at stage IV, the last and worst category in measuring the onrush (or, as physicians so curiously put it, "progress") of the disease. My mother knew how dire her situation was. She just chose not to speak of it.

She did write about it, though. "With daggers lying at the end of my dreams, I [don't] sleep much. . . . I am ill, perhaps irreversibly ill," she noted in her journal as she lay in her bed in Memorial Sloan-Kettering after undergoing that version of a radical mastectomy called a "Halstead." In a Halstead, it is not just the patient's nipple and areola and the breast itself that are removed, but also most of the muscle of the chest wall and the lymph nodes in the armpits, which, in my mother's case, had already been shown to be cancerous. It is a brutal operation, developed at the end of the nineteenth century when excision was the only real tool physicians had. In 1975, for breast cancer as advanced as my mother's, it was still being routinely recommended (it is rarely if ever done today), normally followed up with chemotherapy and, in my mother's case, chemicals to boost her immune system—an approach then in its medical infancy and whose efficacy remains today a matter of dispute among oncologists. In fact, doctors at another cancer center, the Cleveland Clinic, had recommended a far less radical approach. But my mother was convinced that the more that was done, the better her (slim) chances would be, and so she opted for the Halstead and returned to New York.

I do not know what my mother really hoped for or expected during those months, or whether she really believed that she might actually survive. Her two essays on illness are almost *anti*-autobiographical—intentionally so—and in any case were written long after her treatments had ended and all seemed to be well. And after her surgery and during her chemotherapy, she became so opaque to the rest of us, so seemingly encased in her pain and fear, that I felt that to have asked her would have been to sap what little strength she could still muster. But her journals, which she began keeping again quite soon after her surgery, tell a different story. They are punctuated with the repeated notation: "Cancer = death." In one entry, my mother notes without further comment that one of the floor nurses, after leaning over "to swab my papery lips with glycerine," had told her pointedly, "Everyone's got to die sometime."

But what she might have known or at least inferred, whether as probability or as fate, was not the same as what she did. If she managed to confound her doctors' pessimism, somehow she managed to confound her own as well. On the one hand, she could write that she found herself in a state of "leaky panic," and note: "Save my life? No. Prolong it." But at the same time, she systematically set about trying to defy the odds and did everything she could think of to survive. She was not ready to die at forty-two; it was as simple as that. And she believed in her own will, and, grandiose though it may seem, in her own star. Such belief is easy to mock. But everything my mother accomplished, and she accomplished a lot, was undergirded by that belief.

And the salient point is that in an essential sense she wasn't wrong. As her friend, Dr. Jerome Groopman, the chief of experimental medicine at the Beth Israel Deaconess Medical Center in Boston, who is himself a specialist in blood cancers, commented on her decision to me a few months after my mother's death in 2004: "Terrible as the statistics were, there's a sense in which Susan was absolutely right. The statistics only get you so far. There are always people on the tail end of the curve. They survive, miraculously, like your mother did with breast cancer. Yes, her prognosis was horrific. But she said, 'No, I'm too young and stubborn. I want to go for treatment.' Of course, statistically she should have died. But she didn't. She was at the tail end of that curve."

Groopman is a scientist. It is second nature for him to think in terms of statistical curves. In doing so, however, he never loses sight of where on the curve most of his patients are likely to fall. But while my mother must have known something of this, had her doctors told her that stage IV breast cancer was hopeless, I don't know what she would have decided to do. But because there was some small hope of a full remission of her disease, and because, for our different reasons, Bill Cahan and I were both unwilling to tell her just how bad things were, she could find the strength to tell herself that *someone* had to be lucky, and buttress that statistical possibility with a lifetime's experience of believing in her own luck. But it was by no means all magical thinking. She also did what she could, as she saw it, to change the odds.

My mother loved science, and believed in it (as she believed in reason) with a fierce, unwavering tenacity bordering on religiosity. There was a sense in which reason was her religion. She was also always a servant of what she admired, and I am certain that her admiration for science (as a child, the life of Madame Curie had been the first of her models) and above all for physicians helped her maintain her conviction—and again, this, too, was probably an extrapolation from childhood—that somewhere out there was something better than what was at hand, whether the something in question was a new life or a new medical treatment. Soon after she got out of Memorial Sloan-Kettering, she began to search for it. Unreasonable? Probably. But the project of looking itself was immensely strengthening to her during her long, painful convalescence after the Halstead. I remember that it was only when the talk turned to new treatments that my mother's face brightened and the flat, demoralized quality of her language postsurgery became at least briefly energized.

At that time, my mother's companion was a French woman named Nicole Stéphane. In fact, it was entirely thanks to Nicole, who literally refused to take not one "no" but many for an answer, that my mother made contact with Lucien Israël, a Parisian oncologist who was then doing research into immunotherapy as an adjuvant treatment to chemotherapy. Dr. Israël was also working with an Italian colleague, Dr. Gianni Bonadonna, on new combinations of agents to be used for the chemotherapy itself. Dr. Israël looked at the slides Nicole had brought him, and wrote my mother simply, "I do not think your case is hopeless." That sentence was the turning point for my mother. It gave her the strength to continue, and she would subsequently attribute her survival largely to Dr. Israël's care. Perhaps there, at least, was a marriage of magical thinking and reason. The great Danish physicist Niels Bohr used to tell the story of a neighbor who "fixed a horseshoe over the door to his house. When a common friend asked him, 'But are you really superstitious? Do you honestly believe that this horseshoe will bring you luck?' he replied, 'Of course not; but they say it works even if you don't believe in it.'"

But was my mother right to believe? And was Dr. Israël right to hold out such hope to her? Using Jerome Groopman's yardstick, any oncologist could have said what Dr. Israël said to my mother without either lying or betraying his Hippocratic oath, at least in the sense that, indeed, statistically, a few people with stage IV metastatic breast cancer did survive. After all, the Parisian doctor had not told my mother that her case was hopeful or that she was likely to live. But the argument can also be made that what he did, even if technically correct, was to hold out false hope since the main thing that the statistics showed was that the overwhelming majority of people in my mother's medical condition in 1975 died, and died fairly quickly. In my mother's case, what we would today call Dr. Israël's "spin" was a lifeline, a reason to go on. But in another case, one in which the patient was less sure of what she wanted than my mother was? Or were it to serve as a generalized modus operandi for oncologists?

Would what Dr. Israël did have seemed as impeccable?

Yes, hard cases make bad law, as the cliché goes, but medicine is not law and every cancer patient's case is a hard case. I was profoundly grateful to Dr. Israël at the time for what he said as well as what he subsequently did, and I remain abjectly thankful to him to this day. But I am not smart enough to know if he did the right thing. More to the point, I am not sure that most doctors are smart enough to know if *they* are doing the right thing. A scientist, a clinician, and a sage. It's a lot to expect—too much, perhaps.

On another level, though, my mother had few options. The treatment Dr. Israël proposed and that even the New York doctors seemed to agree offered the only chance of survival for my mother was experimental (and the immunological component is no longer as accepted as it would become in the years immediately after my mother received it—another magic bullet in the quest to cure cancer that did not live up to its early promise). For my mother, its effects bordered on the unbearable. The doctors at Memorial Sloan-Kettering agreed to administer Israël's chemotherapy and his immunological prescriptions in New York and, once more, my mother became an exception. Writing of this period, she described how "twice a week I return/haul myself to the hospital and present my opaque body to Doctor Green or Doctor Black [these names, of course, are pseudonyms], so they can tell me how I am. One pushes and pulls and pokes, admiring his handiwork, my vast scar. The other pumps me full of poison, to kill my disease but not me." Her fantasy was bitter. "I feel like the Vietnam War," she wrote. "My body is invasive, colonizing. They're using chemical weapons on me. I have to cheer."

It would be more accurate to say that she *learned* to cheer. Special she might feel, but there is nothing victorious about her tone. Instead, all through the journals she kept during her treatment, she returns again and again to how diminished she feels. "People speak of illness as deepening," she writes. "I don't feel deepened. I feel flattened. I've become opaque to myself." But at the same time, she keeps asking herself how she can transform this feeling. Is there some way, she demands, that she can "turn it into a liberation"?

In retrospect, my mother was painfully acquiring the cultural traits that were simultaneously the privilege and the burden of what she would later describe in her essay "Illness as Metaphor" as her new citizenship in the world of the ill. As the months passed, and as she seemed to be weathering both the toxicity of her treatment and the tremendous psychological adjustment to what she thought of as her new "maimed" self—or, more bluntly put, the damage done to her sexuality from which I do not believe she ever fully recovered—she began not only to hope in earnest that she might survive, but also to fundamentally recast in her own mind what had happened to her. Early on in her illness, she wrote that, much as she might reject it intellectually, emotionally she accepted the old claim of the psychologist Wilhelm Reich—the one that had impelled Norman Mailer, after stabbing his wife, to boast that "I got a lot of cancer out that way"— that cancer was mainly the product of sexual repression. "I feel my body has let me down," she wrote. "And my mind, too. For, somewhere, I believe the Reichian verdict. I'm responsible for my cancer. I lived as a coward, repressing my desire, my rage."

But by the time her treatment was finished, this self-flagellating judgment no longer seemed to weigh so heavily upon her days. (I do not, of course, know what she thought or felt in the hours before dawn when we are all at our most vulnerable.) Instead, my mother began to believe not only that she really might survive, but that living in this new realm—the kingdom of the sick, as she called it—might actually be a context for writing better, becoming a better person; in other words, that there was fulfillment to be had as well as death forestalled. My mother's "default mode" had always been the transcendental, or, perhaps more accurately, that of the exemplary student who also aspires to be the exemplary soul. Don't laugh or smile condescendingly, reader: there are more ignoble ambitions. In retrospect I am not surprised that as she began to recover from the chemotherapy, that was where she again felt both most at home and most in control. And even the illusion of control, even if all it consisted of was collecting information as if for a college paper, was paramount in a situation that, when all was said and done, was out of her control.

"We tell ourselves stories in order to live." This justly celebrated line of Joan Didion's has occurred to me often as I look back on my mother's struggles with breast cancer in the seventies, with the uterine sarcoma in the nineties, and, of course, with the MDS that killed her. For as the years went by, my mother began more and more to think of her survival not as a species of miracle, since the miraculous had no place in the way she thought, nor as an accident of fate or genetics, let alone as a statistical anomaly, but rather as the result of medical progress and also of her willingness to have the most radical, mutilating treatment, which was something many people who subsequently came to see her for advice or referrals for their own cancers refused to do, much to her consternation. As she understood her own story, choosing the milder version of the mastectomy that had been proposed at the Cleveland Clinic would have meant not making the commitment to survival that was required. Real commitment for her was always radical.

As her thinking evolved after this utterly unexpected recovery from metastatic breast cancer, fighting cancer

became for my mother a question of the right information, the right doctors, and the right follow-through, and
above all the willingness to undergo any amount of suffering. I do not mean this in any primitive, public-library
façade, "knowledge is power" sense. It was putting the
knowledge to use that was sustaining for my mother. She
herself became a militant propagandist for more rather
than less treatment—a stance that became harder to sus-
tain as at least some empirical evidence seemed to show
that radical treatment did not necessarily alter patient
outcomes, and that it was the doctors in Cleveland who
had been at the cutting edge of the science. But while
my mother might quote Buckminster Fuller's gnomic
aphorism "Less is more" when talking of aesthetics, as
far as she was concerned when it came to cancer treatments more was always better. That was how she had
survived. How could anyone equally intent on survival
do otherwise? I recall her genuine bafflement over the
decision of an acquaintance of hers not to have a Halstead for her own stage IV breast cancer. "She's just
throwing her life away," my mother said mournfully.

The question of whether this woman was really ever

in a position to be the arbiter of whether she would in fact live or die was not one, at least as far as I know, that my mother ever posed to herself. But how could it have been otherwise? How could my mother *not* have extrapolated from her own experience? No one, not even someone who loved reason (and, more crucially, loathed appeals to the subjective) as my mother did, can be expected to be that rational in extremis. But if it was not subjectivity on her part, I do think there was bravado at work as well. If there wasn't, then how to explain the fact that although my mother was medically literate—after her treatment for breast cancer, *Harrison's Principles of Internal Medicine* was added to the essential books that she kept in her work space—paradoxically, she was also medically somewhat incurious—she for whom curiosity was always a touchstone. It was a matter of conviction for her that great advances were being made both in the understanding and the treatment of cancer, and the advice she gave fellow cancer sufferers was based on that premise. But, assiduous student though she was in any subject that even remotely interested her, she did not follow developments in cancer research, let alone in discoveries in the fundamental biology of cancer, with the care that her intelligence, her considerable layman's knowledge, and even her lifelong interest in science and particular aptitude for biology would have permitted her to do had she really wanted to.

In any case, I am not sure what cause such diligence would have furthered. Would such knowledge have brought her solace or despair? My fear is the latter. For example, if her doctor at Memorial Sloan-Kettering had not conformed to the oncological conventions of the era and instead told my mother in 1975, when she was diagnosed, just how terrible the statistics on survival for stage IV metastatic breast cancer actually were, would she have had the strength of will to go forward with treatment? Reading her diaries after her death, I am overwhelmed not by the force of her will—as I had imagined that I would be since she so prided herself on it—but rather on the depth of her despair. "While I was busy zapping the world with my mind, my body fell down," she wrote in her journal. "I've become afraid of my own imagination."

I have to believe that for her, knowing these concrete

statistics, like fully taking in the realities about the actual scientific and clinical progress (or lack thereof) being made in the effort to understand and treat cancer, would have meant risking letting loose all the devils of her imagination. So in a way, for the sake of her happiness, even of her sanity, I am glad she did not go further than she did in finding out what the state of play in cancer really was. The news was so terrible. The news is still so terrible. As I would find out. As she would find out. The reality, for her, was that it was less a matter of having a sword of Damocles over her head as it was of having it touching her throat. There is such a thing as too much reality.

In any case, our relationship was not one in which I would have been drawn to ask her about any of this. In 1975, when she returned home from Memorial Sloan-Kettering (I had returned home from university to help look after her), she quickly made it plain, though she never came out and said it so bluntly, that there were "no go" areas on the subject of her illness. She did not literally say that she wanted to be told that she would make it, and that the treatment she had received really had saved her life. To the contrary, in words she asked for the truth. But her actual wishes were self-evident to everyone who really cared about her. It was to those that I acquiesced; it was in those that I became her accomplice, albeit with the guiltiest of consciences. But leaving my reading of the situation, the story I told *myself* in order to live, as well as the specific dynamic between us, to one side, I'm not sure I would have said more than I did even had there been a green light flashing invitingly.

It simply seemed out of place, almost destructive, even to ask her if she wanted to know more, let alone to sound a note of caution. This was how I reasoned, anyway, again precisely on Didion's "we tell ourselves stories in order to live" principle. What if, by asking, I inadvertently created doubts in her about whether she really had survived her cancer? What if the Reichians were right and it was how you felt about your chances of survival that helped determine them? I did not believe any of that (nor do I now) any more than my mother did. But I was not prepared to take the risk. Twenty-nine years later, as I tried to understand what it meant that she had MDS, I found I still was not prepared to do so.

III

IN THE AFTERMATH of her visit to Dr. A., my mother could find room for little else but despair. And rightly so, since Dr. A. had left such scant ground for hope. But though she would have been insane to have responded in any other way to the news that she had MDS, the habits of hope survived her loss of it. Almost immediately upon returning home—"from my death sentence," as she put it to me a few days later, before, her face crumpling, she ran into the bathroom—she gamely set about doing what she could to go through the motions of carrying on. Friends needed to be told that she was ill again. Above all, information needed to be collected. Information meant control, did it not? For her, at least, it always had. And control was a prerequisite for hope. Besides, my mother had nowhere else to go. But she did so through the choking haze of her own panic. Disoriented and despairing, she oscillated between a hyper-manic wakefulness and intensity and a bedraggled somnolence. When I would come to her apartment, I felt as if I could feel the ghosts of stillborn screams.

Minutes after returning from Dr. A.'s office, she was on the phone to her friend, Paolo Dilonardo. Minutes after that, she was on the Internet, feverishly looking for information on MDS and AML. Her apartment became a kind of research unit (it had always been more office and library than home), with my mother's assistant, Anne Jump, doing most of the heavy lifting. Remembering how my mother had behaved during her previous cancers, her close friends also began to search online, and were soon e-mailing to Anne the most informative or promising materials or links that they had found online. I say "promising," but that is not exactly right. Given the lack of good news about MDS, "promising" became a relative term. Starkly put, the extent to which the information could be interpreted as giving ground for hope was also the extent to which it was being graded on a curve. For overwhelmingly, what we were all discovering about MDS was just how lethal it was, and just how little hope for anything but a short prolongation of her life, and an easier rather than a harder death (though to this she remained characteristically indifferent) it appeared that my mother could realistically allow herself to feel.

The bad news was unrelenting. Even the terminology itself was terrifying. Take the carefully matter-of-fact and nonalarmist booklet *Myelodysplastic Syndrome* published by the Leukemia & Lymphoma Society, sponsored by the biotech firms CTI and Celgene and mainly directed toward patients and their families and friends. It spoke all too matter-of-factly of MDS also being known as "smoldering" leukemia, or "refractory sideroblastic anemia." "So much for the distinction between MDS and AML," I remember my mother saying with a catch in her voice (the catch in her voice is what I really remember). "'Smoldering leukemia!'" she almost shouted at a friend whom she had called to

report on what she had found so far and who was trying to put a positive spin on the thing. "Don't you get
it? That means leukemia! And what do you think *that*
means?"

Even when outlining possible treatments, it was
above all the toxicities of those treatments—toxicities
of seemingly every imaginable kind, not to mention
those that apparently derived from the disease itself—
that stood out for all of us in the materials we were
finding on the Web, though this was not what we said
to my mother, of course. The operative cliché is "keeping a calm face on things." Keeping a Noh mask on
them is more like it. The reality, in my case at least, was
that I was willfully misinterpreting facts so as to be able
to construe them for my mother if not in an optimistic
way, then at least in a less despairing one. At times, in
those first days, only these upbeat mischaracterizations
could calm her down.

Reality was elsewhere. Most of the time, what we
were finding out about MDS seemed to resemble nothing so much as those "bad news, worse news" doctor-
and-patient jokes that my mother's late friend Joseph

Brodsky had enjoyed telling people who visited him during his many hospitalizations for cardiac insufficiency. His favorite, as I recall, went as follows: A patient comes to see his doctor and the doctor says, "I have bad news: you have an inoperable cancer and only six weeks to live." Devastated, the patient manages to blurt out, "What news could possibly be worse than that?" To which the doctor replies, "We've been trying to contact you for two weeks now!"

There was so much bad news. But the thrust was always the same. Different sources put the matter in different ways. Some read like print versions of Dr. A.; others went to lengths to try to cushion the blow. The Leukemia & Lymphoma Society booklet was one of these. There, the worst news of all was contained in the section called "The Course of the Disease," which in fact was a long paragraph wedged about halfway through the brochure between the section called "Disease Management and Health Problems (Complications)" and the one titled "Emotional Aspects." For once, there was no fluff, and no evasiveness. After a discussion about the need for frequent monitoring of the disease by a physician and the availability of treatments to alleviate symptoms, the (anonymous) authors of the brochure state simply: "Curative therapy is not available for most patients at this time." The only real possibility of cure was a bone marrow transplant that, for suitable candidates, "may have restoration of normal blood cell formation after a successful transplant."

My mother put a double-underline mark under that "may." And when she did this, it was clear that what she was reading was "is unlikely to." In that first week, she shouted that out, too.

But we die as we live. She did anyway. It had been my mother's habit from childhood to underline every book she read. Her underlinings were so extensive, in fact, that to read a book from her library was sometimes impossible since to do so meant reading not so much the book itself as her own "rewriting" of it. With the Leukemia & Lymphoma Society brochure, however, rewriting was out of the question. But even as the weight of what she was reading seemed to be overwhelming her, her ardent bibliomania, or, perhaps more accurately, that astonishing mix of gallantry and pedantry that was one of her hallmarks throughout her life, showed itself in a query on the inside front cover of the brochure. She had noticed that the booklet had no publication date (in fact there are multiple editions). I would have thought the detail would not detain her, but, later, there in my mother's round, plain hand is the query: "2002?" Nor, it seems, did her collector's delight in new words wane right away, either. On another page in the brochure, in the discussion of sideroblasts and sideroblastic anemia, my mother circled the word "sideros"—Greek for "iron"—which was characteristically her way of noting words she didn't know.

Obviously, most of her underlinings were about MDS and AML. The brochure's AML definition struck her particularly hard. It was the "rapidly progressive malignant disease of the bone marrow" into which the MDS eventually "converted." One particularly difficult day during which her despair seemed particularly acute and when neither conversation nor pills had any calming effect, I reminded her that even Dr. A. had told her that she had not "converted" yet (I was always looking for straws to clutch at: from the day we saw Dr. A. to almost the day my mother died that was my default position with her). "Did he?" she asked vaguely. "I don't remember."

Those lapses of memory soon became the norm. She would seem to be completely present and alert during a visit to one of her doctors, but soon after leaving— often it was a matter of minutes—she would insist that she could not recall anything that had been said and would ask whoever was with her to repeat it. But my sense was that she didn't remember these reiterations for very long, either. By the time she would get home, she usually would be unable to tell whoever was there waiting for her much about what had happened, unless she had had a particularly painful or invasive test at the hospital—the bone marrow biopsies were the worst.

If anything, once she got back to her apartment it was even worse. During those first weeks after her diagnosis, she would walk around the flat as if not quite sure of where she was, or of what was solid and what wasn't. Of course, she was not wrong to be disoriented. In "Illness as Metaphor," she could write, not without a certain pride, of her journey from the kingdom of the well to the kingdom of the ill, and her acquisition, as she put it, of that second citizenship. But now, she acted as if it were not the kingdom of the ill she was entering but the kingdom of the dying. She knew. In those early days, *she* knew. It was only later that, for a while at least, she was able to talk herself out of this Promethean knowledge.

Is information, or knowing, power or is it cruelty? Until my mother contracted MDS, I'm sure she would have insisted it was the former. And even after her diagnosis, the habits of information gathering endured, even as her theretofore exceptional memory deteriorated—I believe as a mechanism of self-protection but will never be sure (that subject was off-limits, too). Perhaps that is why, when I first read the underlinings in her copy of the Leukemia & Lymphoma Society brochure after her death, I was not surprised. To the contrary, I felt as if I were following the trail she herself put down so as not to lose herself completely, rather like the breadcrumbs Hansel and Gretel leave behind to be able to find their way home. Except that for her this trail led not home but, if the brochure was to be taken at face value, toward almost certain death—at least in a woman of my mother's age with the severity of what Dr. A. had called, in a rare moment of delicate understatement, and which the brochure had echoed, her marrow cell disturbance.

In fairness to Dr. A., if the booklet was to be believed it seemed that his suggestion that my mother undertake no major treatment before the MDS became full-blown leukemia was very much the received wisdom in Leukemialand. Dr. A. had not been defensive about this, but the brochure certainly was, conceding that, "When a serious disease [sic] is diagnosed and the physician recommends watchful waiting, patients are sometimes dismayed."

My mother was indeed "dismayed." We were all dismayed.

Forgive the sarcasm, reader, or at least try to understand it. The anger I continue to feel, and that I doubt will ever entirely leave me (and, in my experience, is common among people who have watched those dear to them die), makes me unable to resist scoring cheap points at the expense of an informative booklet that, of necessity, is written in lowest-common-denominator language. And I have no good reason, let alone some unprovable suspicion about hidden agendas, that might give me the right to impugn the good intentions of the Leukemia & Lymphoma Society, their corporate sponsors, and the brochure's authors. And yet, rereading the booklet some two years after my mother's death, these undoubted good intentions seem essentially compromised by the refusal to write as if bad news were bad news and despair despair. It is not just the grasping-at-straws aspect of this, although the sentence in the "Emotional Aspects" section, in which those wanting more information about the "social" and the "emotional" are counseled to read another Leukemia & Lymphoma Society booklet, *Coping with Survival,* seems crushingly, unnecessarily obtuse, even for so determinedly upbeat an effort—How about "coping with extinction"? I can almost hear my mother scream. In the end, what really seems unconscionable is the way in which the brochure is written in the language of hope, but in fact offers almost none to anyone reading it with care, as of course my mother did (and I'm sure thousands of other people with MDS have done and doubtless continue to do).

I believe that it was her apprehension of this fundamental disconnect between the brochure's presentation of her disease and the most important information it had been written to impart that drove my mother to underline that "may" in the sentence about stem cell transplants, and also so many other "may"s and "can"s that are inserted, like worms injected into burnished supermarket apples then covered in plastic wrap, into the body of the brochure's text. On one hand, there is all the relatively upbeat talking about "living with the disease," and suggestions that the patient—leaving aside why the reference is not instead to the person—"may" (again!) derive some emotional relief from physicians' explanations and a focus on what the brochure calls "the treatment ahead and the prospect of improvement." On the other is the real news—that is, the *bad* news—sandwiched between the language of the laboratory and the language of self-help. So admirable in other contexts, here the language of hope becomes grotesque. By mischaracterizing the reality, it inadvertently betrays those it seeks to help by effectively infantilizing them and speaking to them as if they can't see through all that equanimity and poise to the terrible things they are, or soon will be, experiencing.

One example (in the "Need for Treatment and Treatment Approaches" section), bracketed between the Biology 101 tone of the information that "cytogenetic evaluation can be helpful in reaching a conclusion about the diagnosis" and the meaningless banality of "Living with a serious disease can be a difficult challenge," lies this nugget of unvarnished reality: "In the very small proportion of patients who are under 50 years of age with a severe form of myelodysplastic syndrome, intensive radiation and/or chemotherapy followed by allogeneic stem cell transplantation can be considered."

Here is the worst news being given in the language of the best case. Again, I do not pretend to know what the best alternative would be. The brochure is meant to be informative and comes not only with contact information for the Leukemia & Lymphoma Society and the National Cancer Institute, and a list of suggested further readings, but also three lined pages on which the patient or loved one can write notes. But surely, even in a medical booklet, there are ways of imparting hard information, information that hurts, that will make you weep, in tones other than that of Pollyanna. No one is asking for a John Donne poem as an epigraph or an enclosed CD of a funeral march. But the gap here between language and reality is simply too great, and is actually a disservice to most patients and their loved ones, and, I suspect, even for physicians and nurses as well. No, truth probably is not power—much as we all might wish it otherwise—but that does not make it any less indispensable to understanding. It may be appropriate to "redirect" a small child who is upset about something. It is not appropriate to "redirect" an adult cancer patient.

But that begs the question of what, for my mother, the consequences were to be of such understanding. To take on board the reality of her disease, to regain at least control over what she would choose to do next, she urgently needed to know what her blast counts were—that is, how many leukemic cells were *already* in her bone marrow even though she did not yet have full-blown leukemia. And she needed to know her white blood cell counts, her red blood cell counts, and her platelet counts, because how low these counts were usually correlated with the progression and severity of the disease, with the rule of thumb being the lower the count, the worse the news, just as the higher the number of blast cells, the worse the news. But if the news was very bad, as we all feared it already was, and soon would probably get a great deal worse, then was not the assumption that somehow it could then be "used" in a way that would materially improve my mother's situation itself a grotesque, Pollyannaish conceit? Was it not, when all was said and done, magical thinking disguised as practical research—the old human fantasy of dominion over death, but in which we now substituted the acquisition of information for the philosopher's stone and the alchemist's potion, all on the false premise that with that information there would be something new and transformative that could be done?

Question: What was my mother looking for? Answer: What the condemned always hope for—a commutation of sentence, a reprieve.

In John Gay's *The Beggar's Opera*, a play that my mother loved and at one time wanted to direct (will my head be filled, to the day I die, with the list of things in *her* head that she had hoped to accomplish, or even had "on the drawing board," but that remained undone at her death?), Captain Macheath is finally brought to the gallows to be hanged. But then there is an intervention. Addressing the beggar (one of the characters who is also the author of the play), the player (another of the characters) protests. Is Macheath really to be hanged? he asks the beggar. Yes, the beggar answers. His play, he says, is meant to be realistic. The player is indignant. An opera, he exclaims, must end happily. For a moment, the beggar considers, then assents. "Your Objection, sir, is very just," he tells the player, "and is easily removed," and then he shouts: "So, you Rabble there, run and cry A Reprieve! Let the Prisoner be brought back to his Wives in triumph."

What do you call a reprieve in Leukemialand? A remission.

But why bring an eighteenth-century work of art into this, no matter how much your mother loved it?

The answer is that somewhere I think the player's expectation about an opera has, however irrationally, become the collective expectation of many modern people, including my mother, and, for that matter, including me, about illness. It may not be something people admit to; many may talk starkly about their own death, almost as if they were trying a jacket on for size (I do that). But somehow a fundamental disconnect has now arisen between the reality of death and the reality that one has to die of something. For unless one dies in an accident, is murdered, starves to death, or is killed in war, one presumably is going to die of some disease— more likely than not of cancer given the considerable progress that has been made during the last thirty years with heart attack and stroke and also given the fact that people are living longer. How to reconcile the reality of human mortality with the reigning assumption in the rich world that every disease must have a cure, if not now then sometime in the future? The logic of the former is the acceptance of death. But the logic of the latter is that death is somehow a mistake, and that someday that mistake will be rectified.

Perhaps this is why the "War on cancer"—the phrase was Richard Nixon's when he signed the National Cancer Act in 1971—is a metaphor that continues to make sense to most people in 2007. On a recent broadcast of the ABC evening news, the reporter led his story about improved cancer cure rates by insisting "this is one battle we are starting to win." But is winning the war on cancer what is really meant, or, instead, winning the war on death—that chemical immortality my mother had once lamented to me that we were both, though probably just barely, going to miss?

And if the underlying goal is immortality, or at least the extension of life beyond anything imaginable today, then how could the war metaphor *not* be appealing? After all, in war one side is defeated. My mother's essay "Illness as Metaphor" is to a large extent an attack on this militarization of the struggle with disease, and ends with the plea to give such images "back to the war makers." But she subscribed with her whole being to a far deeper assumption regarding contemporary medical research—at least as it exists in the public mind—which is that cures will eventually be found for most if not all diseases. That faith had sustained her since the days when, at least retrospectively, she had come to terms with her breast cancer. It continued to give her strength when she was stricken with the uterine sarcoma in the late nineties. And when she first realized she was ill again, she had hoped to be able find solace and strength in it once more, even though realistically, with MDS, and at her age, the bad odds of surviving any advanced cancer had become prohibitive.

Even now, I am astonished by the extent to which she succeeded. What I do not know is whether her success in this was a blessing or a curse.

IV

In the immediate aftermath of her diagnosis, my mother at times seemed to oscillate between a hollowed-out somnolence and a sharp, manic busyness that occasionally edged into hysteria, and at other times seemed almost incongruously rational and calm. It helped enormously that her apartment was always filled with people. As she had gotten older, my mother had found it increasingly difficult to be alone (only when she was deep in a piece of writing was solitude even remotely bearable). Now that she was once more ill, even the briefest interregnum of solitude was intolerable to her, and those who were close to her soon organized a kind of rota to make sure that there was always at least one other person in her apartment and preferably more than one. The English writer John Berger once wrote that the opposite of to love is not to hate but "to separate." Certainly, that is what my mother thought—and what could have been a more understandable reaction in a woman who barely knew her own father who died when she was four?

Long before she became ill again, this anxiety was becoming more and more crippling. She would grow anxious whenever a visitor would get up to leave, and she would often ask Anne Jump to prepare lists not only of her own complicated travel plans but the plans of those close to her—me, Paolo Dilonardo, Annie Leibovitz, her on-again, off-again companion of many years, and a few others. After a meal, she would often propose an errand or two—a trip to a bookstore or a record shop, or at least a final cup of coffee (she was a social drinker, but no more). Now, of course, there was no question of her being left on her own. Even surrounded by people, her anxieties often overwhelmed her despite the Ativan that her doctors insisted she begin taking. And yet, characteristically, my mother was surprised by how anxious she felt, and once insisted to me that, without denying how terrified she was, she couldn't really believe she was having anxiety attacks. When I responded that I thought she had been an anxious person for quite a long time, she neither agreed nor disagreed. Instead, she said the idea surprised her and she needed to think about it.

In reality, her mood cratered, then lightened, then cratered again—an increasingly vicious cycle. But for all that it was an emotional roller-coaster ride, what I remember most vividly from that time is how eerily normal it soon came to seem. There was even an incongruous, almost communelike atmosphere, a giddiness that while obviously only a half step from hysteria and grief was also strangely exhilarating. My mother's own behavior probably explains most of this: the rest of us soon grew accustomed to taking our emotional cues from her (or trying to, anyway). And while she obviously was not as interested as she had been before her diagnosis in what was going on around her, and at first made no effort to try to write (though, like most writers when they are not writing, she talked about writing all the time), she was still more connected than I ever would have predicted given what must have been going on in her head.

As I recall it, the only visible reflection of the noises and the silences of dread in her mind was the occasional wild grimace that would suddenly contort her features only to disappear just as suddenly. She still sat in her kitchen in the mornings, holding court behind the scarred wooden table that she had bought from a thrift shop shortly after coming to New York in 1959 and that she had never been able to part with even though she had gotten rid of almost every other object from that time of impecunious promise, discomfort, and enchantment. And she still was almost as eager to talk about what she had read in that morning's newspaper, or about an upcoming concert or movie, or about the book she had been reading the night before, as she had been before she had known she was ill again.

I use the word "known" with considerable misgivings. One of the questions that I cannot drive from my mind is whether my mother had had any inkling before those blood tests and bone marrow biopsies delivered their catastrophic verdict that there was something deeply wrong physically. She certainly would have had ample cause to consider the possibility of this since in the year before her diagnosis, she had a number of medical problems, the worst being a severe bout of pleurisy that led to a partly collapsed lung. More worryingly still, as Anne Jump later told me, Sookhee Chinkhan, my mother's housekeeper, had been asking her for months with steadily deepening alarm why she was regularly getting bruises all over her body—bruises that because of their location could not possibly be attributed to bumping into a piece of furniture or some other domestic accident. My mother had been noncommittal, and, Sookhee Chinkhan told me later, would usually insist on changing the subject.

But what I wish I knew is why something that alarmed my mother's housekeeper appears not to have alarmed the doctors who had treated my mother for her uterine sarcoma and to whom she still went for regular follow-ups. These examinations were extensive and often included flushing out the port that had been implanted in a vein in her neck after her surgery so that the chemotherapy could be administered without having to puncture a new vein with each treatment. Of course, I do not know what her doctors said to her, but I do know that my mother never understood there to be any urgency. Nor, whatever they said, did they communicate it to her in a way that she really took in the fact (again, I do not know what they said: I only know what my mother heard) that some of the chemotherapy drugs routinely given those with uterine sarcomas lead to leukemia in a number of them. In relating this, I am echoing my mother's surprise, which she expressed frequently in the last months of her life, usually in a tone of voice far softer and more indistinct than the one she normally employed. She never contacted any of these doctors nor did any of them contact her, and their silence was a subject of such bleak and unfathomable regret to her that she, who was comfortable enough with her own indignation and thus more prone to saying everything she thought than to censor anything, in the end could barely stand to mention the subject.

What my mother did do was ask Stephen Nimer, the head of the leukemia service at Memorial Sloan-

Kettering, who became her principal doctor shortly after her initial diagnosis and, before too long, her friend as well, whether knowing she had MDS a few months earlier would have made much of a difference to her prognosis. And I believe she derived a certain cold consolation from his reply that it would not have changed things very much. What Stephen Nimer could tell her with great confidence was that tests on the particular cytogenetics of her disease that he had rerun after she presented him the results of Dr. A.'s blood tests and bone marrow biopsy led him to conclude that her MDS *was* the result of the chemotherapy she had received for the uterine sarcoma. But beyond asking Jerome Groopman and a number of other physicians who treated her if they agreed with Stephen Nimer, my mother did not pursue the subject, nor, as I say, did she attempt to contact the doctors who had administered the chemotherapy for the sarcoma. At the time, I felt that she simply could not bear to know any more about what had happened six years earlier. Instead, almost from the moment she met Stephen Nimer, she talked of little but the possibility, however remote, of cure.

Still, I continue to ask myself whether she actually did know she was ill or, at the very least, suspected it. Even at the time, I was not alone in this. With hindsight, we are all soothsayers, and there was much talk in my mother's intimate circle about how badly she had looked in the previous six months, how something clearly had been wrong, and how surely one of her doctors should have noticed that all was not right with her. But as these conversations petered out—and in the end, what difference did it make now?—the same plaintive question would finally be posed out loud: "Why hadn't *she* noticed?"

For me, the force of this question derived less from the foreshortened perspective of hindsight and more from a piece of information that at the time I preferred to keep bottled up inside myself. For I knew something about her behavior during her previous cancer that she preferred to keep to herself, as far as I know telling only her greatest friend, Paolo Dilonardo, her companion during that period, and me. I did not want to capitulate to this knowledge; I did not want the guilt that came with knowing what I knew, and yet *not* having paid enough attention to her episode of pleurisy or checked with Sookhee Chinkhan who was probably the only person whom my mother was completely at ease with physically in the last part of her life, about the state of her health. To think about this would have meant thinking of my mother as old—something I had never done (knowing something and thinking about it are hardly identical). For if I had thought of her as old that would have meant confronting, *really* confronting, I mean, the prospect of her death. It was a folie à deux, I suppose: the thing she wouldn't do was the thing I couldn't do.

"In reality," John Berger once wrote, "we are always between two times: that of the body and that of consciousness." For my mother, whose pleasure in her own body—never secure—had been irretrievably wrecked by her breast cancer surgery, consciousness was finally all that mattered. I believe that if she had been offered the possibility of an immortality that consisted of nothing but consciousness, that is, of continuing indefinitely to know what was going on, even if it was the science-fiction immortality of the disembodied head, she would have accepted it with relief and gratitude—perhaps even with appetite. With her, this had absolutely nothing to do with admiring the world. She once joked with a friend that she wanted to live as long as possible "just to see how stupid it gets." But her fear of death was always far, far stronger than anything else—stronger even than her profound, and in the end inconsolable, sense of being always the outsider, always out of place.

And yet the story I had learned about was one in which she had courted death in a way that normally you would associate only with someone whose attachment to life was flimsy rather than tenacious. For her work, she was willing to dice with extinction. The story proved that. At least as she told it to me, the details are straightforward: In 1998, she had closeted herself in Bari, Paolo's hometown, in order to finish work on her novel *In America*. Thomas Mann once wrote that a writer is someone for whom writing is harder than it is for anyone else, and certainly my mother felt that as acutely as any writer I have known. *In America* had been a daunting project, the result, perhaps, of her sense that *The Volcano Lover*, her previous novel, had been the best thing she had ever done. And for a long time, the book had not gone well. But there in Bari, which had long been a refuge for her, after so many false dawns she later told me, she realized to her own delight that she knew how to finish her book. "Nothing can stop me now," she told me she remembered thinking. And then, only a few days later, she began first to urinate blood and then began to feel a constant sense of bloating. "Of course I knew I was ill," she told me, "and I was virtually certain I had cancer again."

"But you stayed on to finish the book," I said. "Nothing was going to stop you, not even your own body." We were sitting across from each other at that scarred table in her kitchen. It was two years after her surgery for the uterine sarcoma and a year after her chemotherapy had ended. She was facing the glass door that gave out on the Hudson. I was facing her.

But there was no need for her to reply and no real point in her doing so. And there was nothing sensible for me to say. Was I supposed to reproach her for her decision? If there had ever been an appropriate time for that, it was long past. And in any case to have done so would of course have been about me, not about her.

Is it too corny to say: she was what she was? Throughout her life, my mother oscillated between pride and regret over her sense of having sacrificed so much in the way of love and pleasure for her work or, as she almost invariably referred to it, *the* work—a conceit that she would occasionally mock herself for in some of the more self-lacerating entries in her journals but to which she nonetheless remained fiercely attached and from which I don't think she ever really tried to divorce herself. *The* work had to be served, and served at any price. Since her adolescence, she had let nothing stand in its way. I wish she could at least have said "in *her* way." I certainly always believed that she served herself badly by the self-objectification in which such rejection of the personal pronoun involved her. But that was psychology—and I am not sure I was right or that anyone can know what another needs—whereas this was existence itself. What I had not understood before she told me about what happened in Bari in 1998 was how far she was willing to take it—she who was so afraid of extinction. So I said nothing. As I remember it, I smiled, then, for once at a loss for words, she smiled back, and that was the end of it. We never spoke of it again.

But after she was diagnosed with MDS, I again wondered if she might not have made a similar decision, at least unconsciously, during the previous year. Obviously, the symptoms of something being badly wrong were probably not as clear-cut as they had been five years earlier. But they were bad enough. Why had she ignored all those bruises? Not to tell me was one thing. But why had she not at least told Paolo Dilonardo, the one person in her life to whom she confided everything? Even Paolo heard about the bruises for the first time only after the MDS was confirmed.

But perhaps this is all pointless—a quest for meaning where no meaning is to be found, or, worse, an attempt on my part to turn my mother's death into something over which she had some control. What in reality was due to the defects in her genes and the deferred result of poisons pushed into her system in order to prolong her life is somehow easier to accept if it was instead due to the defects of her psyche. It's easy to condescend to Reichian or New Age fantasies of why people get ill and why some die and a few recover when it doesn't involve you or someone you love. And for a while I was tempted by the thought that her death was, indeed, something she somewhere wished for—thanatos exacting its revenge. There is such consolation in unreason, which in all likelihood is why the world will always be a charnel house. Better to think of her as a suicide than a victim of some defects in her indifferent genes.

But that is precisely what she was, although even the word victim is probably a distortion. Surely human insignificance is at least as much of a mystery as human existence. The great British scientist J. D. Bernal writes somewhere that there is "the history of desire and the history of fate and man's reason has never learned to distinguish between them." More mundanely, there is one strong reason that, for all my doubts and anxieties, leads me to believe that my mother was not in fact aware before her diagnosis that something was wrong. And it is the worst reason I can imagine: her desperate panic on learning she was once again in cancerland and that this time the odds against her were worse than they had ever been.

Nothing could change that, not the daily routines in my mother's apartment or the intermittent gaiety that was not the smallest of her accomplishments in that catastrophic time. The fact remained that everything we who were closest to her were all discovering about MDS seemed to darken the picture. I think that at different times, each of us had to stop reading what was on the Internet. But because life spares you nothing, I think of that time after my mother's death when I found this notation in her workbook for "Illness as Metaphor": "leukemia: the only clean death from cancer, the only death that can be romanticized."

Alas, no. As we were finding out during the brief period between my mother's diagnosis and the time her treatment began in earnest.

It was a time of endless phone calls to doctors and people who were in touch with other doctors, and to acquaintances and even to acquaintances of acquaintances who had some experience with leukemia, some advice to give, or some new doctor or treatment to suggest. On the phone with these people, my mother would often appear to be cheerful and invariably seem lucid. Her questions were probing, and she took endless notes. Again, the student in her came to the fore. But afterward, it was as if a schoolroom blackboard had been wiped clean and all that remained was an arc of streaky white chalk where the lesson had been. My mother would stare dully, almost quizzically, at the notes she had taken. Often she would then look at Anne Jump, or me, or another of the small group of her "accompany-ers" as I came to think of us. And even if she was aware that no one had been listening in on another line to the conversation she had just had, she would nonetheless ask to be reminded of what had been said.

To say that we were all worried about her immediate mental state does not begin to describe the anxieties those close to her were feeling. Obviously, there is no comparison between the sufferings of a person who is ill and the sufferings of those who love them. But I think there is something similar about the helplessness you feel as a friend or a relative. Some people thought that she had gone mad—to which my own response at the time was that I doubted this was the case, but, if it was, then she was more than entitled. I certainly wondered if I was going mad. To which I was certainly *not* entitled.

In the meantime, the information accumulated. The straight-A student in my mother could focus on that. Looking back over her notes, I find mostly a matter-of-fact record of what she was hearing or getting from the Web. In the beginning, this mostly consisted of definitions of MDS, AML, and their various subsets, and possible treatments, above all the 5-azacitidine that she already had been told might prolong her life for some months but did not offer the possibility of a cure or even a remission longer than a few months, and the various forms of stem cell transplants that in a minority of patients did offer the hope she was looking for. Almost as common are notes about mortality rates, durations of remission. One entry notes that with relation to her particular form of MDS, "survival: 1 in 7." Looking back, I wonder if she realized how wildly optimistic that actually was for her specific situation.

But survival was her goal, and that never changed from the moment of diagnosis almost to the hour of her death. But while she knew she had a deadly illness, good student though she undoubtedly was, this did not make her any less lost, as almost all patients are, in the thick fog of the alien language of medicine and biology, and in the thicker fog of passing from being an autonomous adult to an infantilized patient—all need, and fear, and pain. Words like "apoptosis," "myeloid" and "lymphoid" leukemic cells, "autologous" and "allogeneic" stem cell transplants, and "clonal" disease are noted and then defined. But off the page, as she tried to summon the will and gain at least the minimum of familiarity with her own disease needed to decide what to do next, what use was she to make of all this? From the notes, it would seem that she had taken it all in. A clonal disease referred to all cells coming from the same stem or parental cell. Apoptosis in the context of MDS meant forcing the immature blast cells to self-destruct.

And autologous transplants were those using identical stem cells either culled from one's own body or derived from a sibling who is a perfect DNA match, while allogeneic transplants come from unrelated donors who are a more approximate match genetically.

But what was she to do with this information? Some of her notes on various doctors who had been recommended to her highlight the impossibility for a nonscientist of making sense of much if not most of what she was being told. The scientific papers were largely unintelligible while the mortality rates were all too intelligible. Even my mother, so supremely confident in her own ability to "work up" subjects and master information, found herself incapable of following what she was being told. I felt much the same way, as if I had suddenly found that I had become a functional illiterate. There was all this information, but it was in a foreign language *and*, when translated, it generally turned out to be bad news.

In any case, information is not knowledge. I don't think that I ever really understood this—understood it viscerally, I mean—until this period in which we all floundered around in my mother's beautiful apartment, searching the Web for a miracle that was not on offer, much as she told herself otherwise and those who loved her chose to suspend their disbelief, whatever they knew in their dreams.

V

WHEN MY MOTHER was at her most disconsolate,
she would often say, "This time, for the first time in my
life, I don't feel special." It was that sense of being special—luck is too weak and above all too impersonal a
way of putting it—that had allowed her to both get
through her two previous cancers and, retrospectively
at least, to view the fact of having survived the disease
as somehow more than a statistical accident or the luck
of the biological draw. It was not that she wasn't frightened, let alone that somewhere, in some deep, irrational
part of her being she believed that she was "meant to
live," or any such mystically inflected megalomaniacal
nonsense. But she *did* believe that she was "special" in

exactly the way so many artists do. "If I don't believe in my own work," she once said to me after one of her books had received a particularly disdainful review from a writer who made much of how seriously my mother took herself, "why should anyone else?"

I do not believe that even a person of a different temper from my mother's would have been detached enough to have simply attributed her survival to such impersonal factors. Honestly, I doubt that there are many people capable of such dispassion. If you were supposed to die, and you live, in defiance of practically all the experts' predictions and against all odds, how can you not attach some meaning to what has occurred? How, above all if you struggled to find the right doctors, and braved the most gruesome treatments, can you really say to yourself that none of this really had much to do with why you were still walking on the earth rather than dissolving under it? It is hard enough for any cancer patient to really resist the idea that some failure on his or her own part brought the illness on. After all, Reichian explanations of psychological repression causing cancer have in our time tended to give way to explanations based on one's having eaten the wrong foods, the basis of such self-blame, and the assumption that the cancer patient is in a deep sense the author of his or her own disease is still very much in the air.

But say you do get beyond all that and you do survive. That survival feels like a miracle no matter how much you may know intellectually that in all likelihood it isn't. Miracles aside, at the very least, again, even to the most skeptical of temperaments, it is bound to feel that it has some meaning. In other times, and other mind-sets, this is the stuff out of which religious conversions were fashioned. In Christianity, in particular, it is an old trope. Think of the story of Saint Ignatius Loyola—the warrior surviving his terrible wounds and, when he had done so, forsaking his worldly life to found the Jesuit order.

My mother experienced no conversion. Her atheism was as rock solid when she died as it was in the heady time before her first cancer when the frailties of the body were as unreal to her as old age, even if a few of those close to her tried to inject religion into her burial service, and even, after the burial was over, took to chanting prayers over her grave that would have meant less than nothing to her. But I believe that her experience of surviving confirmed for her that sense of specialness that had sustained her from childhood forward. Contemptuous of the false optimism of the age—something she associated with the deep America she came from and which she both feared and despised—my mother nonetheless shared it, if only unconsciously, where the question of illness was concerned.

I also think that it would have been superhuman for her not to have felt she deserved at least some credit for having survived, if only because of how much she had been prepared to suffer in order to do so. In this, her own sense was that her positive attitude had been a factor in her having lived (rather than in the literal, biochemical sense of a positive attitude somehow strengthening the immune system or helping the chemotherapy's effectiveness). To be sure, this kind of optimism was not so very different from the "official" optimism of the American cancer establishment in its constantly repeated public pronouncements that tremendous progress was being made in cancer treatment and that, in the words of a recent director of the National Cancer Institute, Andrew von Eschenbach, within fifteen years it was quite likely that cancer would be treated as a chronic disease, like AIDS, rather than as an illness from which you were more than likely to die. The packaging of this optimism made my mother wince, and when she read the triumphalist accounts that appeared in the media about "winning the war on cancer," "turning the corner on cancer," and the like, she would usually roll her eyes or make some derisive comment. But in the end, she was as much a believer in it as anyone—even if, to be honest, I'm not sure that she was entirely aware of being so.

Sometime before she was diagnosed with MDS, my mother, who was vertebrally indifferent to competitive sports, became interested in the bicycle champion Lance Armstrong. What drew her to his story, of course, was the fact that he had been given hardly any real chance of survival after being diagnosed with metastatic testicular cancer a dozen years earlier. And yet not only had he lived, but Armstrong had gone on to win Tour de

France after Tour de France. My mother died before he won his record-breaking seventh Tour, but I am certain his victory would have elated her. And his own account of having set out to "beat" his cancer by finding the right doctors who would administer the most cutting-edge treatments very much mirrored her own sense of what she had done when diagnosed with breast cancer. She, too, had refused to settle for the treatment on offer; she, too, had searched far and wide for a specialist who could provide a treatment that would change the odds and allow her to survive, even if the conventional wisdom suggested that survival was not a realistic possibility; and she, too, had spent most of the rest of her life informed by the sense that if you did these things, you had a real chance of not dying.

For two people as different, even in their way of expressing themselves, as my mother and Armstrong, the similarities in their thinking are astonishing to me. Recently, after he had set up a foundation to lobby for more resources for cancer research and treatment, Armstrong appeared on a CNN special broadcast to publicize the project. When he was asked by an interviewer if, after having been diagnosed, he had ever despaired, he replied, "You have moments, for sure, moments of weakness where you think, I'm going to die or perhaps I'm going to die . . . I was totally committed, totally focused and I had complete faith in my doctors, in the medicine, in the procedures."

Watching him—my mother had already been dead for over two years—I realized with a start that it could have been my mother answering.

Reading her diaries, I am now aware that this was not in fact the way that my mother had experienced her surgery and subsequent treatment for breast cancer as they were taking place. But it was the way that she came to remember it and it was this "rewriting" that informed the way she lived from that time forward. For my mother, her own story was emblematic of the rationality of hope. As she construed it, her medical trajectory had gone from lethal diagnosis, to medical pessimism, to the search for doctors who did have hope to hold out (in my mother's case, Dr. Israël in Paris), to agonizing but nonetheless potentially lifesaving treatments, to cure. You did not give in to cancer, you fought it, and if you fought hard enough and, above all, intelligently enough, there was a chance that you could win.

Obviously, I do not mean by this that my mother was foolish enough or self-obsessed enough to believe that cure was a foregone conclusion. Nothing could have been further from how she understood her situation. But the *possibility* of a cure, even if only in a small minority of cases, had been enough to give her hope at the time of her breast cancer treatments and enough to inform her thinking thereafter. And the way that she had come to understand what she had gone through was that some hope was enough, even if it was only the possibility of a treatment that would induce a period of remission of the disease. The grimmer news about cancer she pushed away, I think. Instead, she employed what I can only describe as a kind of "positive denial." That sense that in ignoring bad news she could somehow stay strong, keep going, and, above all, keep writing was something that marked her as a person. In retrospect, though, I realize that, obsessed with death as she was, this positive denial was at a deep level the denial of death itself.

This was not always the way she spoke. To the contrary, for my mother the difference between remission and cure had itself become blurred after her breast cancer. As she had once exclaimed, the brute fact of mortality meant that on the most basic level all human beings are never more than in remission from death. And yet on another level, when she spoke of remission she was banishing death, at least enough to go back to work, back to planning the books she would write in the future, back to collecting books and prints, back to traveling. It was almost remission as synonymous with coming back from the dead—a Persephone who would never need to return to be ferried across the river Styx.

There is a story that on the scaffold, the famous courtesan of the court of Louis XV, Madame du Barry, begged her executioner for "just one more minute of life." My mother was physically almost foolhardily brave and she was far too dignified a person to have ever begged anyone for anything—least of all another minute of life. But she was willing to sacrifice anything except that dignity *for* more time in the world, and by the time she was diagnosed with MDS had proved it not once but twice. She thought the science backed her up, believing that medical progress in cancer research was progressing so rapidly that if, say, she could obtain a remission for a couple of years, there was at least a chance that new experimental treatments would be developed in the interim that might then be used to induce another remission, and so on. Call it scientism, but it was this that finally informed her sense of what was possible.

I am painfully aware that described in this way my mother's views could seem like the expression of faith rather than reason. And on one level, perhaps they were. But her faith in reason was not only, well, unreasonable. As my mother saw it, she had survived her breast cancer by taking this approach, and, far more recently, a great friend of hers who had been diagnosed with a severe case of another blood cancer—CML, or chronic myelogenous leukemia—had done the same. Edward Said was determined to live in large part because, like my mother, he felt there was so much more he had to write. And like my mother, Said was indifferent to the question of how much physical suffering he would have to endure to do so. And suffer he did. In the last two years of his life, Said's treatments made his stomach swell up to the size of that of a pregnant woman in her third trimester. And he suffered indescribable pain. But as my mother repeated over and over again (he had died some months before she was diagnosed with MDS), "look at all the work he got done with those extra years."

A person is already somewhere on the lower rungs of hell when they wish they had been lucky enough to be diagnosed with the disease that killed Edward Said. And yet that is precisely what my mother felt; indeed, what she said—bitterly and often—after she was diagnosed with MDS. For what we had learned was that with MDS and unlike, say, CML, there were absolutely no treatments that could induce a remission long enough for there to be any realistic possibility of some further medical advance coming along to induce a further remission, and so on. Indeed, there was no question of any remission at all. Rather, someone with MDS or AML who wanted to fight to survive had only one option: to try for a complete cure, that is, an adult stem cell transplant in which, in effect, the mortally afflicted blood system would be destroyed and a new one introduced to replace it. In doing so, the doctors had to first literally destroy the body's immune system. But otherwise, to quote one of the medical Web sites that my mother visited during those first weeks after her diagnosis, treatment could only focus on "alleviation of symptoms, reduction in transfusion requirements, and improvement of quality of life."

"Quality of what?" my mother asked incredulously as she read me the sentence over the phone shortly after she had come across it. Then I heard her weeping. "Say something," I kept thinking. But I could think of nothing to say. Perhaps some people transcend themselves when a loved one becomes ill, become demonstrative where before they were inhibited or withholding, and cheerful where before they were morose. But even if that's the case, I was not able to become one of them. Instead, I said nothing. My mind was a doleful blank.

Fortunately, there were those in my mother's immediate circle who could provide her with what I could not. The ways in which they did this varied. Her more

"New Age" friends could, with perfect sincerity, bring her pretty rocks and crystals and speak of their healing powers. Her more maternal friends could cook for her. Her Buddhist friends could write her that she was within a "protected circle" and that meant she would pull through. Her more cheerful friends could try to overwhelm her panic with the charm of their conversations and the warmth of their reassurance. Her more political friends could distract her with talk of politics. Her Christian friends could send her images of saints and write that they had said intercessory prayers.

But diversions only helped a little. My mother was not a believer. She had a longstanding Wildean appreciation of the Roman Catholic Church but nothing more. Her Jewish origins were of scant interest to her. Certainly she had never had any truck with New Age or Buddhism. What she wanted was for someone to say about her MDS what Dr. Israël had said to her in 1975 about her metastatic breast cancer: that her case was not hopeless, that there was something that could be done. And yet from everything that she was reading about her disease, almost nothing could be done. She wanted at least to be in the realm of possibility, the realm of hope. Without it, her days were unbearable.

Very soon after we went to see Dr. A., I realized that for her one of my principal roles in her struggle to live had to be to offer reassurance that it was at least possible that she *would* live. I am in no sense flattering myself or claiming for myself an importance I did not have to say that my mother wanted not just reassurance about her chances, but reassurance from me: What did I think? Was she in good enough shape for a bone marrow transplant? Was the idea that one's biological age could be different than one's chronological age something that she dared take seriously? Was the progress being made in adult stem cell transplants enough to make her undergoing one realistic? These were the questions that she would pose to me—as if my opinions had any scientific value!

I answered as best I could. What I mean by this is that I gave the answers that I believed she wanted to hear, the answers that would give her the strength to go on. And it was so clear that what she wanted to hear was good news and nothing else. Of course, sometimes even giving the right answer did not pierce her despair. I think I did right. But I did it ineptly. Inside, I was shutting down, almost as if, instinctively, I realized that I could not handle my own emotion as well as hers, as if also I could not tell her these things and be aware of myself enough to know whether or not I myself believed them. At the time, this shutting down seemed like an inevitable choice. Looking back, though, I am by no means sure it was the right one.

By this, I obviously do not mean that I wish I had become hysterical in her company or worn my feelings on my sleeve, let alone that I believe that I should have told her of my own doubts about her chances. But I do think that by keeping the darkness out of my thoughts, I somehow let the cold in as well. Rationally, I am all too well aware that guilt over what one did not do for someone who died is an inescapable emotion. I don't think it's an inappropriate one, either. But it is also an impossible emotion because the guilt comes no matter what you have or haven't done. To live without guilt after the death of a loved one, a person would have to accede to literally everything the other person wanted.

And what that really means is living one's entire life in attendance of the other's death since there is no way of being an emotional Jain in relation to others. The Jain may decide to always walk bent over sweeping the road so as not to inadvertently kill some tiny insect in his path, but deferring completely to another person is, if anything, an even more impossible project. For such deference would render one without personality—without the very qualities, in other words, upon which one's relations with the other person are grounded.

One of Jerome Groopman's favorite phrases is Kierkegaard's remark that while life can only be understood retrospectively, it must be lived prospectively. Often, when I think of my guilt over all the things I didn't do for my mother—whether through unwillingness or inability, though actually I don't think that much matters—I think of that phrase. Sometimes it helps, sometimes it doesn't. Of course, I know that on the most basic level, this entire way of thinking is not only useless but absurd as well. One *cannot* live one's life bending to another person's desires on the basis of some actuarial conclusion that one likely will outlive them. And yet I don't think I am alone in wishing I had been able to do so, no matter how weird or stupid it may sound. But when she wept, and she wept often, I did so little.

I do not think this was mainly because of my own fear of death (although it must have played some role). Rather, for me at least, coping with accompanying my mother in her own struggle—something I was determined to do, and, rightly, it never occurred to her that not only I but also her immediate circle of friends *wouldn't* do—meant becoming something of a stranger to myself. The description that occurred to me at the time was psychological intubation. I wanted to take up as little psychic room as possible. In being in some sense part of my mother's emotional life support, I found *myself* to be on emotional life support. That still feels appropriate to me, but looking back I still wish that it had been otherwise. Had it been, I doubtless could have given more. At least I would have had the means to have given more. Again, I very much doubt the specific nature of my relationship with my mother is of great significance in these regrets and afterthoughts. To the contrary, on those occasions when I have talked about these feelings with other people who have lost parents, they mostly express similar regrets, no matter how different their temperaments are from mine, or their parents' from my mother's. But I have never asked any of them if they were sure that they should have lied, as somewhere I always felt that I was doing.

MY MOTHER had always thought of herself as someone whose hunger for truth was absolute. After her diagnosis, the hunger remained, but it was life and not truth that she was desperate for. I hope I did the right thing in trying to give it to her, but I will never be sure. But she was clear about what she wanted and to the extent that I am consolable about the role I played, this is what consoles me:

She was entitled to die her own death.

VI

DURING THE MONTHS I watched my mother die, I was increasingly at a loss as to how I could behave toward her in ways that actually would be helpful. Mostly, I felt at sea. Of course, this had much to do with some of my own grave failings as a person (above all, I think, my clumsiness and coldness). Had I been a better person, doubtless I would have had at least a somewhat more intelligent apprehension about what I should have done. But even to put my own failings at the center of this is a species of vanity. The crux of the matter was that my mother's illness and, as soon became clear, the cumulative side effects of her treatment, increasingly had stripped her both of physical dignity and mental acuity—

in short, everything except her excruciating pain and her desperate hope that the course she had embarked upon would allow her to go on living. I knew that for her the physical agony she was undergoing—and I am not being even slightly hyperbolic when I use those words—was only bearable because of this hope and that therefore my task had to be to help her as best I could to go on believing that she would survive. For me to have behaved in any other way would have meant saying to her, in effect, "your sufferings are for nothing: you gambled everything on a transplant, but you've lost."

There is a Jewish saying, "Just as it is an obligation to tell someone what is acceptable, it is an obligation not to say what is not acceptable." Never for a moment, during the course of my mother's illness, did I think she could have "heard" that she was dying. Bedridden in the aftermath of her bone marrow transplant, her muscles soon so flaccid and wasted that she was unable even to roll over unaided, her flesh increasingly ulcerated, and her mouth so cankered that she was often unable to swallow and sometimes unable even to speak, she dreamt (and spoke, when she could speak, that is) of what she could do when she got out of the hospital and once more took up the reins of her life. The future was everything. Living was everything. Getting back to work was everything. And though her mind was fuzzy from chemicals—"chemo brain," as cancer patients call it—and she was often disoriented and wild-eyed, seemingly in focus and out of her head, she counted the days until she might be released. The emblem of this was that, after her transplant, on the wall opposite her bed in her room in the University of Washington Medical Center, she insisted that we put up a sheet of paper where each day we would mark the number of days that had elapsed since her transplant. These numbers marked the first days of her new life, she would say.

Her emphasis was always on this fresh start that she was about to make. It was a point on which my mother was adamant. She wanted to change things, she kept telling those of us vigiling with her in Seattle, not to mention the doctors, physicians' aides, and nurses who would stop to talk with her; she wanted to shake things up. When she was finally able to return home to New York, my mother said, she would write in a different way, get to know new people, do some of the many things she had been meaning to do and stop doing still more of the many things that no longer gave her pleasure. She told me at one point that she was tormented by the amount of time she had wasted during her life on what she called her "Girl Scout–ish" obsession with doing "worthy" things. Now, she would take advantage of the new lease on life that the transplant would give her and do the things that really mattered to her. Did I agree? she asked, and as she did so her eyes seem to bore into my face. I agree, I said. Later, back at my hotel and for the only time between the first night after I had accompanied my mother to see Dr. A. and the day, some weeks after her death, when I finally broke down, I wept. But my stupefaction was almost as great as my grief. I kept thinking, "She really does not know what is happening to her. She still believes that she is going to survive."

During my mother's illness, I very consciously decided to take no notes. Perhaps no writer can escape the sliver of ice in the heart that is one of the professional deformations of their craft, but to the extent I could, I wanted no "writerly" distance to separate or protect me emotionally from the reality of what was going on. So my memory is all that I have to rely on and doubtless it is faulty: the Rashomon effect and all that. Looking back, her death seems inevitable. But did it seem that way at the time? I cannot be sure. I am almost certain that once she went to Seattle for the transplant, my mother believed she was going to live. There was even a moment at the University of Washington hospital when she had told Paolo Dilonardo, whose own father had died of MDS, that his father had not survived because he had not really wanted to live (this was true: Signor Dilonardo had declined treatment), but that she thought she had a chance at surviving because she desperately wanted to go on living.

It would be easy to say that, on the deepest level, my mother did not understand what was happening to her. But I'm not at all sure that's right. Yes, her chances of survival were small. But I remember thinking at the time that I simply did not have the right to be more pessimistic about her chances than her doctors were. And they were going ahead with treatment, presumably in the belief that it was not futile, and that she was not wrong to hope. Obviously, I knew that not all the doctors shared this view. My mother had started out with Dr. A., after all, and he certainly gave her no reason to believe that there was much that could be done. But Stephen Nimer at Memorial Sloan-Kettering and Jerome Groopman did not seem to believe that there was no sense in her fighting even if she wanted to. Who was I to insist that my dread was more relevant than their expertise?

In any case, I never allowed myself to actually transform the dread that had become my default mode emotionally into the concrete, clearly articulated thought that no, my mother would not survive her illness this time. I wish I could say that I did this because somewhere I believed that she would make it, as so many of her friends did (after my mother's death, I got a number of letters from old friends of hers expressing sorrow, yes, but more emphatically their disbelief that she had not lived). But the truth is that I was afraid to feel anything, not least because I was so acutely aware of what my mother wanted from me—to believe that she would once more overcome the odds and recover from her disease. To do that, I had to not think. But I soon discovered that this "not thinking" was insufficient. If I was to believe, if I was to play my part in my mother's revolt against death, I needed a model.

AT A LOSS at first (I was so numb for so long), what I finally did was to take my cues about how to be helpful to my mother from her doctors. On the immediate level, they had the authority and the skills to lift her at least temporarily out of her despair whereas I did not. On a more profound level, they could offer hope that was grounded in something objective, not simply my mother's desperate wish or that of her loved ones. I do not mean to idealize science here. I am well aware that my mother's doctors, too, had an emotional stake in helping her survive including, or so I have always assumed, anyway, the investment of their own ego in the struggle. Nor am I unaware of how much so-called heroic medical treatment for diseases for which there are no good cures of necessity, for doctor and patient alike, on a certain level represents the triumph of hope over experience. Had I been the one pushing my mother to be treated, I imagine that I would now be subject to a different variant of guilt (for the survivor, guilt is the constant, though). Instead of regretting that I did not help her enough in her fight, I suppose that I would feel I had pushed when I should have let her die, if that was what she wanted. But my failing was that my own ambivalence about the choice she had made often rendered me almost mute.

That was where my mother's doctors came in. They had the words that I needed. I remember thinking that if I observed them carefully enough, perhaps I could learn how to talk their talk. I am not much interested in sports, but the metaphor in my head was that of a pinch hitter in baseball. What I hoped was that I could be a *rhetorical* pinch hitter, filling in until I, or one of the other people in my mother's immediate circle, could get a quick appointment with Stephen Nimer or get Jerome Groopman on the phone so that they could work what did seem like nothing short of magic and reel her back up from the black well into which she had fallen.

How they did this I never understood, not from my mother's first consultation with Stephen Nimer until the morning of her death, when he stood at her bedside, staring gravely down at her, his hand holding hers, as she drew her last breath and then drew no more of them. On one level, the calming, and sometimes even the emboldening effect of what her doctors would tell her seemed almost entirely irrational since she was hardly being told that her chances were very good. To the contrary, when pressed Stephen Nimer would be very frank with my mother about just how terrible her MDS was. It is true that he never allowed himself to be drawn out on whether he personally thought my mother would survive or not (though she repeatedly tried to get him to do so, and asked me to ask him on a number of occasions as well). Instead, he would reframe the question, and in doing so, or so it seemed to me, let the hope back in. My mother would almost always take a deep breath, shake her head, hair flying, and ask questions concerning the next step Nimer wanted to take in her treatment. They would go on from there, with my mother growing visibly calmer with the passing minutes.

To be sure, the successful dynamic between them

depended to a large extent on my mother not digging in her heels and simply repeating the question about whether Stephen Nimer thought she would survive or not until he was forced to reply to her either by his words or by his silence. But she never did anything of the sort, nor did she ever inquire of me whether I had in fact posed the question to Nimer myself as she had asked or how he had responded.

OF COURSE she did not want to know the answer. *Of course* somewhere she knew perfectly well that the answer she would have got would have sent her into an emotional freefall from which there would likely be no coming back. But it was more than my mother's fear or instinct for psychic self-preservation that determined the trajectory that these consultations with Stephen Nimer would follow. For in large measure, I always felt, it was Nimer himself who determined this outcome. Somehow, whether it was through force of personality, long experience, or psychological acuity, or some combination of all of these, Stephen Nimer managed to make the question "unaskable" on some deep level.

There are doctors who, for all the deep respect they have for great physician-scientists like Stephen Nimer, are critical of this approach. After my mother's death, Diane Meier, a physician at the Mount Sinai Hospital in New York who is one of the pioneers in the movement to improve palliative care for terminally ill people, offered a very different view. "It's so difficult," she said. "As a physician, you don't want to impose your quantitative, Cartesian view of probabilities on an individual person who says, 'That's probabilities, that's not me. I'm a fighter. I want that thousand to one chance and who are you to say that it's not worth it?' Whose life is it anyway? The result is that, as doctors, we end up through that kind of thinking becoming unwitting participants in a folie à deux with patients and family of caving to the desire to live, because it is respectful of the patient and who she or he is and their perception of the right way to live, while realizing, in the other part of your brain, that there's essentially no chance that this is going to help, that it's definitely going to cause harm and side effects, that it's hugely expensive out of the public trough, and it is a very wearing kind of cognitive dissonance."

Meier's tone seemed more despairing than critical. She spoke of "the denial, the kind of winking that goes on, where, yeah, we all know the patient's going to die but we're all going to pretend like there's hope, so we're all going to go through these rituals because that's what we believe that the patient wants. In the meantime the patient is watching the doctor, who is offering this treatment, and clearly thinking to himself, if the doctor didn't think it would work he or she wouldn't offer it, but what the doctor's not saying is that the odds are minute and that he is trying to be responsive to the needs of the patient for hope. It's like a minuet. It's surreal."

It *is* surreal. But what is the alternative? Stephen Nimer frames the issue quite differently. It is not that he has any illusions about his own powers. As he put it to me, "I'd have to be an idiot to think everything I do works. I mean, where have I been the last twenty years? I'm not afraid to fail. And of course I know that I'm not going to save everyone."

But for Nimer, the essence of being a doctor was

doing everything possible for his patients, even if it meant trying experimental therapies where the chances of success were not high. This was exactly what he did after my mother's transplant failed and she returned from Seattle to his care at Memorial Sloan-Kettering. My mother still wanted to fight; it was all she had left, and all that was allowing her to keep some tenuous hold on sanity. And Nimer was prepared to fight, recommending an experimental drug called Zarnestra. He did so without illusions. Later, he would tell me that "there was a possible scenario in which things would have worked out for Susan. But of course there were many scenarios where things would not work out. But the bottom line was that she still wanted to fight for her life and in my mind, there was a way for her to get better. If I hadn't believed that, if I had thought, 'There's no way,' I wouldn't have given her the Zarnestra."

For Stephen Nimer, there was no minuet. His approach was consistent from first to last. As he said to me as we were leaving his office after my mother's first consultation with him, "I do what I can." After my mother died, when I was first attempting to write about what had happened, I asked Stephen Nimer how he saw what he had done during these first encounters. "You told her the absolute truth, and yet you made her feel better," was what I actually said to him, before confessing that both his approach and its effect had always seemed completely mysterious to me.

Nimer, as always, was matter-of-fact. "There are ways to say things," he said. "When I first met Susan she repeatedly told me that she was 'in freefall.' While I didn't really know precisely what she meant, I thought she meant that things were out of her control, that she felt she had no way to turn the tide against the further deterioration in her health. So rather than quote statistics to her, I felt it important to focus on the real possibility that she could get better. I didn't see why, or what good it would have done to quote a bunch of numbers to her. Whatever I would have said wouldn't have changed the numbers. She needed to know that things were not 'hopeless.' In any case, I've always felt that if I tell someone they have leukemia, I don't have to also stress to them that they have a fatal disease. Susan knew that. They all know that. But with her, as with all my patients, I feel that before people get to the time of dying, people want to have some hope, some meaning, and, if it's at all possible, the sense that there's at least a chance that things can get better."

Had he taken his lead from her? Stephen Nimer did not answer directly. "She was not ready to die," he said. "As far as seeking treatment, I knew from the first time I met her that she would rather die trying. There was also the feeling of loss of control and of wanting to regain control. And I did think that there were things to do for Susan. The transplant had a chance to work. Had I thought differently, I wouldn't have made the recommendations I made. But when I told Susan that there was a chance, I meant it. And if there is a chance, and if what one of my patients wants is to go for it, then I feel my duty as a physician is to try to make that happen. It was not that Susan just wanted to be told that she had a chance to be cured. She *did* have a chance to be cured. Let me tell you: When I first meet a possible stem cell transplant candidate, and my assessment is that there is really no chance for success, I am clear in my recommendation. I care a lot about my patients and don't want to mislead them. If they are my patient, and not merely seeing me for a second opinion, I want them to know that I will take care of them no matter how things turn out. While I get emotionally involved with what my patients are experiencing, I still need to keep an important and significant distance, so my medical judgments are not colored by emotions. Susan drew me in closely, due to the strength of her personality and her intellectual power, but I never felt that I made emotional decisions. In fact, we understood each other very well, and it was easy for me to carry out her wishes.

"Susan told me from the outset that she wanted me to do everything she could to save her life, and so we could go straight into a discussion about what she wanted and what the plan would be."

I do not believe for a moment that it was easy. But that is of little significance. Stephen Nimer could not save my mother's life, but what he did do was save her sanity during the time that remained to her. By the time she got to the Fred Hutchinson Cancer Research Center in Seattle, which Nimer believed was the best place for her to have the bone marrow transplant, she, too, had come to believe there was a chance. Indeed, she had come to believe it so strongly that when, sometime during the full day devoted to admissions procedures at "the Hutch," its clinical research director, Fred Appelbaum, dropped by to remind my mother of the poor survival statistics he had told her about when she had gone to Seattle earlier for an initial consultation, she was devastated. That evening, still completely devastated, she kept repeating, "Why would he tell me such a thing?" Later Appelbaum would tell me that the purpose of his visit wasn't to "'remind her of the poor survival statistics,' but rather to make sure she was going into the procedure with her eyes open." At the time, however, the truth was that I had no idea why he had said what he said. But I was so worried about my mother's state of mind that I immediately tried to make up an explanation that, or so I hoped, would take the sting—that is to say, the reality—out of Appelbaum's words. That first day in Seattle, which might have passed relatively smoothly, in fact was haunted by what my mother took to be Appelbaum telling her she would not survive. And the next morning was not much better. By sheer luck, I remembered having read somewhere that the Hutch had been taken to court, accused by the relatives of some patients whose loved ones had not survived their transplants of not having warned them of how small their chances of survival had really been. With no basis whatsoever for saying anything of the sort, I told my mother that I was *sure* that the only possible reason Appelbaum could have said what he had said was that the hospital's lawyers must have insisted that patients be reminded of the risks they were incurring in coming to the Hutch for their transplants.

To say that I persuaded my mother is to badly overstate her reaction. But the explanation, bogus though it doubtless was, served to put a "bottom" on her resurgent panic. The freefall was halted. She could believe she could make it again. In fact, until months later, when she was actually told by her doctors at the Hutch that the transplant had definitely failed and that her leukemia had returned, the only times she really seemed to doubt that she would survive were when she recalled Appelbaum's words. At those times, too, I would trot out my little playlet about the hospital having had to

get all lawyered up (the phrase amused my mother; I'd
gotten it from a John Grisham novel I'd read in a hospital waiting room soon after my mother had been
admitted). And she would start to question what I was
saying—how could she not have done?—but then seem
to stop herself. One more victory for the Joan Didion
line about telling ourselves stories in order to live, or, in
this case, to believe we will go on living.

VII

IN ANY CASE, I had nothing better to offer her than stories. It is not as if I even had the right to an opinion concerning my mother's chances of survival. I could echo what Stephen Nimer or Jerome Groopman or Fred Appelbaum said, though I certainly must have gotten a good bit wrong. I could embellish, or, as I did in response to Fred's caution to my mother, I could try to soften the blow. But beyond that, while I could swim in that sea of death alongside my mother and her doctors, they knew where they were going and I did not. The biographical irony of the fact that, from childhood, I was formed—or do I mean deformed?—by my readiness to form opinions and stick to them was not lost on me. Doubtless, it was a deserved and overdue comeuppance. But to dwell on that fact, while it might have been morally instructive to me, was of no use whatsoever to my mother. To the contrary, whether or not I had the intellectual right to do so, what she wanted above all from me was the same thing she wanted from everyone who committed themselves to her from the time of her initial diagnosis, through her treatment, to her death. And that was to buoy her up, to tell her over and over again versions of the same reassuring mantra: "you're going to survive, the transplant is going to work, it's not hopeless."

In some ways things were easier back in the days when doctors routinely lied to their patients about their prognoses, and sometimes about the actual nature of their illnesses as well, and when there was no Internet for a patient or a loved one to turn to in order to uncover the bad news for themselves. The relatives of those who were truly fearful and for whom death was literally unbearable could and often did collude in such lies, and, in doing so, buy some measure of serenity for the dying person. That is what Simone de Beauvoir and her sister did for (or to: I am not wise enough to say) their mother as she was dying. As Beauvoir recounts so movingly in her memoir *A Very Easy Death*, having been told by doctors and family that she had peritonitis rather than cancer, the elder Mme Beauvoir literally, as her daughter put it, was "there, present, conscious, and completely unaware of what she was living through . . . she rested and dreamed, infinitely far removed from her rotting flesh, her ears filled with the sound of our lies."

Obviously, there was no question of treating my mother in this way. Cancer was for her an old companion: she was a veteran; she knew too much. More to the point, she was loyal to the activity of acquiring information as one is loyal to a faith. Therein lay my mother's most deep-seated conviction about herself— her belief in her ability to take in and understand facts and then to face them. As she often said, that sense of herself had served her well as a writer and she believed that it had also helped her survive her two previous cancers. She had coped, she thought, precisely by playing to her intellectual strength—that is, through having been assiduous in learning everything she could about both her illnesses and their possible treatments. In some odd way, for my mother information had become synonymous with hope: the more you knew, the better your chances of cheating death once more.

Denial, then, was not on offer. But this time, information was more likely to be undermining than sustaining, and for her to have contemplated the unvarnished reality of her situation would have meant staring without respite into the mouth of the void. Of course, on one level my mother knew this. That was why it was so critical for her to find a way to look away and yet to feel as if she were not looking away. Of course she knew. That was why she kept repeating in those first weeks after her diagnosis that this time the facts seemed so terrible, the odds so stacked against her. In someone with a different temperament, as Stephen Nimer had pointed out to me, this might have eventually led if not to acceptance then at least to resignation. But my mother was not wired that way, and people don't change nearly so much as our contemporary culture that so fetishizes self-help and self-transformation might lead us to believe. Some of her doctors in Seattle, I later discovered, were surprised and not a little undone by her rejection of any consolation, whether spiritual or familial. But no one who knew her more than casually was surprised that my mother, who had never reconciled herself to any essential thing, would die unreconciled to her own extinction and that hers would end up being the opposite of an easy death.

But despite what she discovered about MDS, it was literally only in the last few weeks of her life after the transplant had failed and she had returned from Seattle to Memorial Sloan-Kettering that she essentially gave up trying to find ways to believe there were rational reasons for her to think she would survive. It was an impossible balancing act. For it was as if she were trying to remain loyal to the idea of the truth and to the supremacy of the factual yet at the same time looking for ways to deny what these facts suggested.

As a result, what conversations I had with her about her prognosis soon became almost lawyerly exercises. And like a lawyer making an argument for a client with the weakest of cases, I found myself grasping at some minor point, or emphasizing some faint possibility as if it could be construed as being a medical norm. Perhaps an even better analogy would be to a politician. The spring and summer of 2004 was a period in which the extent to which the Bush administration had "cherry-picked" the intelligence in order to find a pretext to go to war with Saddam Hussein became fully known. I remember coming home after a long period sitting in my mother's apartment trying to make the case that despite the statistics she actually stood a decent chance of surviving her MDS and rather numbly turning on the evening news. The expression "cherry-picking" was being used repeatedly. That was what I was doing, I thought, there was no doubt at all about that. That was fine. My real fear was that I wasn't doing it very well, and that my impersonation of an optimist was so transparent that I was actually of very little use to her.

But whether or not I was in fact up to the task, I never had the slightest doubt that this was the role that my mother wanted me to play in her illness. There were people with whom she talked about death, but I was not one of them. What she wanted from me was an adamant refusal to accept that it was even *possible* that she might not survive. Every day seemed to bring new illustrations of this. From her first meetings with Stephen Nimer where he managed so seemingly effortlessly to restore her equilibrium, through the journey to Seattle and the horrible preparations for the transplant—preparations that involved basically destroying her leukemia-compromised immune system with massive doses of radiation—to the three months after the transplant during which she suffered illness after illness, infection upon infection, all the time still trying to believe, or, as I think, still actually believing that she was going to survive, my mother looked to those of us who were with her not just to keep telling her that she was right, and that there was a real empirical basis for hope, but also to give her the reasons why this should be the case. That neither I nor anyone else in her circle had any right to an opinion, that, to the contrary, our factual opinions were quite literally valueless, never seems to have occurred to her.

For me, the contrast between the assurance I felt I had to not just feign but incarnate (if I couldn't at least in the moment make myself believe as well, it wouldn't work) when speaking with my mother and the sense of being an ignorant fool I had when I would speak with her doctors would have been comical in almost any other context. In the morning, I might be visiting my mother in her hospital room and, though she might be covered in sores, incontinent, and half delirious, tell her at great and cheerful length about how much better she seemed to look/seem/be compared to the day before. Then, that afternoon, I might e-mail one of her doctors because I had read on one Web site or other some promising new treatment for MDS and wondered whether it might help in my mother's case. Exhibiting a patience I did not deserve, the gentle reply via BlackBerry would usually not be long in coming. It was always one version or another of either "despite what you read, it actually doesn't apply in your mother's case," "you've misunderstood what you read," or "what you're reading in the press is hype and the results that are described are actually nowhere nearly as promising as the story you've forwarded suggests."

And these overhyped stories were almost all I had in the way of material to make the case my mother wanted me to make. It is perhaps fortunate that such stories were (and of course still are) to be found on practically every news site from the BBC to the Associated Press to Reuters. It made doing what I felt was expected of me, well, doable. But if I am being honest, I do not understand how my mother was able to reconcile her immense respect for the depth of knowledge of the physician-scientists who were caring for her with the idea that, for example, anything I said to her about her chances was of any significance or that these stories were occasions for hope. What I do know is that desperate as my mother was for hope, she was never content with those expressions of it that could be understood solely as a declaration of love on my (or anyone else's) part. In the midst of all her bad fortune, that at least was her good fortune. The luck of the genetic draw had given her that fatal predisposition to cancer, but at least she was lucky enough to be able to take the love part for granted and assume that those who loved her would devote themselves to her as well.

I wonder if she even realized that one does not always follow from the other.

If love was stable, the case for survival was volatile. Perhaps that was why it was only when the argument that her situation was not hopeless was presented as being based on scientific facts that she could be even partially persuaded that there was, indeed, some reason not to lose hope. Anything else, no matter how loving, was for her not just unhelpful but counterproductive— the doorway to despair, the doorway to her death. She craved objectivity. The pathos of it was that she demanded this objectivity from me and from others who didn't have nearly enough knowledge to be objective. All we had, in the end, was feeling. And it was not enough.

If, for example, someone said to her, "I feel you're going to make it," as several of her more New Age or otherwise mystically inclined friends did either in person or through e-mails and letters, my mother would respond indignantly, often exclaiming, "How can you possibly know that?" Far from being reassured, such sentiments, even though of course she knew them to be well meant, not only infuriated her, but actually deepened her sense of hurtling toward extinction. At those times she would often explain in a pedantic tone that soon spiraled into panic how few people survived MDS and how bad her chances of being one of them really were. "Read the statistics," she'd say, "read the statistics."

That hapless friend who had made the suggestion that a crystal would bring good luck was rebutted with a shouted, "Don't you understand? Luck has *nothing* to do with this!" Then, rummaging through the printouts of articles on MDS from medical journals and from the National Cancer Institute Web site, my mother began to numbly recite the catalogue of reasons that would, as she put it, "persuade any sane person" that she was unlikely to survive her disease. "It's a question of the cytogenetics of my disease," she said finally—she was white-faced and almost breathless by then—"and they're terrible!"

At such times, no one around my mother, least of all me, seemed to know what to say. Looking back, I wonder if there is any silence worse than the silence of the

sick room. It is the silence of that horror-stricken intuition that in a cancer ward, at least, the real and the catastrophic are often one and the same. And of course it
is also the silence of impotence, of the powerlessness of
feeling to change anything, of the vanity of human
wishes. You find yourself hoping, and yet you know
there is no empirical basis for such hope. The words
form, but fail to emerge when you open your mouth. In
your head, there is a voice screaming, "Say something,
do something!" But there is nothing to do and everything that seems possible to say, at least to someone
who wants to be reassured of something that you don't
have the basis to reassure them of, either has no bearing on what is really going on or involves you in pure
fable making—a species of nannyspeak. In effect, you
find yourself saying a slightly more sophisticated version of "there, there, it will be all right." But that is a
lie. It will not be all right . . . as somewhere you know
perfectly well, no matter how much you deny it to
yourself or others, or even set about intubating yourself
psychologically to the point where you don't even think
it at three in the morning.

So often, what was said was precisely the wrong thing, the thing that made my mother weep. Early in her illness, when she was still at home in New York and doing relatively well physically, my mother received a gift from a Buddhist friend that was accompanied by a note saying that she was convinced my mother was inside a (Buddhist) circle of protection and that all would be well in the end. It was a sentiment, nothing more, harmless, well intended, if perhaps somewhat ill-considered as well. But it drove my mother wild. "This is *grotesque,*" she said as she tossed the letter onto the kitchen table in her apartment. Then, looking wildly around the room, she added, "Somehow someone forgot to tell my genes." After that, she burst into tears and then fled toward her bedroom, not to come out for hours.

On these occasions, it was usually only when she finally spoke to one of her doctors that she would regain some measure of equilibrium. Perhaps this was one of the few benefits of that profound (and probably inevitable) infantilizing asymmetry at the heart of what goes on between doctors and patients. In this context, at least, Stephen Nimer at Memorial Sloan-Kettering or John Pagel, an attending physician at the Hutch in Seattle, were less physician-scientists than shaman-scientists with the power to somehow mitigate the unthinkable. And it is all very well to deride that aspect of the relationship between doctor and patient, to speak of how patronizing or objectifying it is, but I am by no means sure there is a way out of the dilemma or even that more candor from the doctors would have been any sort of improvement. For the sad reality is that without the doctors' power to infantilize, which in this context meant to lull and reassure, not condescend to or lord it over her, my mother would have gone mad months before she died.

I do not mean to imply that my mother was not grateful for the love she received from those she was close to. She was immensely grateful. Nonetheless, the stark truth is that this love was no consolation to her as she fought so desperately for her life. And in the end, those of us who loved her failed her as the living always fail the dying, for we could not actually *do* the only thing she really wanted, which was to stave off extinction for just some time longer, let alone give her what I'm afraid is all too accurately called a new lease on life. Only her doctors could do that. So she clung to them, as a shipwrecked sailor to a spar, for as long as she possibly could, even after the bone marrow transplant had failed, almost to the last days of her life, while the rest of us looked on helplessly. In the end, when she could not even turn her body and when there was only sleep or pain, we could only bring her newspapers she could no longer read and music she no longer wanted to hear, or rearrange the bedclothes, or hold her hands, or roll her over, or listen to her as she rambled—sometimes comprehensibly, more often not—or tweak one of the drips when they stopped, or call the nurses.

There was nothing easy about my mother's death, except, literally, her last few hours. It was hard, and it was slow—sometimes the days of her dying seemed to me to actually be taking place in slow motion—and in the process it was not only my mother who was stripped of her dignity.

VIII

If only my mother hadn't hoped so much. But to say this is to posit the impossible. Throughout her life, my mother had been incapable of doing anything else but hope, hope *in extremis,* and against all odds if need be. I do not mean to imply that she was a cheerful person. Quite the contrary, she was almost always dueling with depression. This was clearest immediately after she woke up, when, in an effort to shake off her despondency, she would talk, about anything and at breakneck speed, as if to overwhelm her mood with meteor showers of verbiage. And yet, paradoxical as it may seem, even the ways in which she parsed her own despair could themselves appear like a subspecies of hope. I only realized this fully when I saw on the first page of one of her journals, written in the immediate aftermath of her breast cancer surgery, the sentence "Despair shall set you free." At first, I assumed she was making a morbid joke, but, reading on, I discovered that she had been entirely in earnest. "I can't write," she noted, "because I don't (won't) give myself permission to voice the despair I feel. Always the *will*. My refusal of despair is blocking my energies."

Described in this way, my mother's exhortation to herself to "give in" to despair becomes a new project of self-transformation, even of self-improvement, almost in the same way that her self-assigned reading lists and itineraries were such projects. But how could it have been otherwise? My mother's refusal of despair in its conventional, paralyzing sense, and, more than that, her sense that whatever she could will in her life she could probably accomplish as well (except in love: there she thought herself bereft of any gift and did not believe the will of any use at all), had served her so well for so long that, empirically, it would have been madness on her part not to have made it her organizing principle, her true north.

When she was young, the strength of my mother's hope and that steeliness of her will that became the source both of such pride and such rue to her—for her, the two almost always went hand in hand—had seemed the only way to survive. "I lived on a high horse," she writes in one journal entry, "without saddle sores." And she told me more than once that she believed that hope and will had been all she had to see herself through her alienated childhood, get herself out of the Southwest and on to the University of Chicago, where, at seventeen, she agreed to marry my father after knowing him for a little more than a week. Seven years later, that same sense of being able to remake her life no matter the obstacles— and not just remake it but also to make version two, or three, or four better than their predecessors—had given her the strength to extricate herself from the marriage.

BERKELEY, Chicago, Cambridge, Mass., Oxford, Paris, and then finally New York: these were the places to which the winds of hope had carried her (they were also the places, as she sometimes would say, where in her imagination she already lived when still an adolescent in the arroyos of Tucson, Arizona). Always, there was a fresh beginning, a new first act. Writing in one of her journals of her arrival in New York, she reports feeling that "like smoke evaporating, my failed marriage wasn't there anymore. And my unhappy childhood slipped away also, as though touched by magic."

For someone in love with the past, or, more exactly, who identified with the great achievements of the past and their architects—in a sense, she was her admirations—my mother was surprisingly untroubled by nostalgia. The two great, besetting regrets of her life were not having accomplished more in previous years and not having known how to be happier in the present, where, by her own admission, her private life was a source of sorrow and frustration. From a political and, increasingly, an ecological standpoint as well, she had no great hope that the world would get any better, and, at the very least, the strong intuition that it would probably get a great deal worse. But these were intellectual conclusions, not visceral ones. And as the saying goes, "Pessimism of the intellect, optimism of the will." The simple truth is that my mother could not get enough of being alive. She reveled in *being*; it was as straightforward as that. No one I have ever known loved life so unambivalently, and I am almost certain that had she lived to a hundred, as in the last part of her life she so often said she hoped she would do, instead of seventy-one, nothing except the loss of intellect would have made her any more reconciled to extinction. She was with the great Peruvian poet César Vallejo when he wrote:

> *I'd like to live always, even flat on my belly,*
> *because as I was saying and I say it again*
> *So much life and never! And so many years,*
> *and always, much always, always always!*

Obviously, my mother knew she would die. She was under no illusions that she lived in an outtake of *Star Wars*. But that is where for her, as, I suspect, for so many others, whether the ill themselves or their loved ones, the modern difficulty came in. For you don't just die, as Simone de Beauvoir points out in her beautiful memoir, "from being born, nor from having lived, nor from old age. You die from *something*." But instead of dying from the particular something, cancer, that had her in its gun sights since she was in her early forties, she survived not once but twice. From a strictly scientific point of view, there is nothing all that surprising about a case of breast cancer that has metastasized into the lymph system being beaten back by the chemotherapy and then recurring a decade, or even two or more decades, later. But it would be humanly unrealistic, and demand not just an abandonment of hope but also a repudiation of experience, for someone who should have died of her cancer but lived and then survived for many years to continue to tell herself that her remission was just as likely to end at twenty years as at five—the scientifically misleading but generally accepted "cutoff point" after which cancer patients are at least led to believe that they are more likely than not to be in the clear.

MY MOTHER came to being ill imbued with a profound sense of being the exception to every rule. Again, she was hardly alone in this. On a certain level, all modern people who are not utterly beaten down by experience early and whose good fortune is that their tragedies come later in life feel this way. To feel otherwise (whatever you may know intellectually) is to put oneself at odds with the dominant message of our culture, manifest in everything from our advertising to our politics—the one that says "me, Me, ME," and tells you lie after lie: "this product is made for you," "elect me and I will do what you want," "you can be whatever you want to be," "you are the world." My mother did not even have a television set, but she was not made of moral and cultural Teflon, either. But to understand an illusion is not to rid yourself of it, and she was fond of citing the English writer John Berger's idea that we live in a society in which each person is encouraged to aspire to be, or thinks of himself or herself as being, not so much exceptional (that *is* an artist's vice) but as having been granted an exemption from pain, illness, and even death itself.

Did my mother know how deeply she had been affected by this species of wishful thinking? Before her first cancer, I am not sure that she did, but after it, despite the fact that she had survived against all odds, and even if only in some banked and rarely expressed way, I believe that it was the principal thing she knew. Her obsession with time, her ever-increasing need for distraction—"When I can't write, I can't stop reading," she remarks in one of her journals; "I'm sucking on a thousand straws"—all seem to me part of this flight from nothingness. And yet if she no longer could believe herself exempt from the humiliations of the flesh, there was a way in which she came to believe that she would indeed be the exception. And she was willing to dice with her own life informed by this sense, as when she postponed both diagnosis and treatment for her uterine sarcoma so that she could finish her novel *In America*.

I do not mean to imply by any of this that she was hopeful in the sentimental *Gone with the Wind*, "tomorrow is another day" sense of the term. Nothing could have been further from her way of seeing the world. Her experience of being treated for breast cancer had given her a graduate education in pain. She knew what she would undergo when she went back home, was operated on, and began chemotherapy. But bearing pain, which she who could be so divalike and unstoical about trivial things did so stoically, is not the same as believing that one's death cannot be put off once again, and that, while one is going to die, one is not going to die of *this* thing, *this* time. That was why, virtually from the moment that she was diagnosed with MDS, I thought my role was to lead her once more to the same belief that she would survive this as well and that there would be more time.

She thought the world a charnel house . . . and couldn't get enough of it. She thought herself unhappy . . . and wanted to live, unhappy, for as long as she possibly could. That unhappiness haunts me still, even if the waves of guilt that wash over me periodically are by now old comrades. Czeslaw Milosz says somewhere that it is possible that the only real memory is the memory of wounds. Is it possible that the deepest feelings we have for the dead we loved is guilt? I hope not. But I'm almost certain that it is one of them. I feel guilty, therefore I am? It would be a good motto for visitors to gravesites.

What misery there is even in the most ostensibly

successful, fulfilled lives! Some months after my mother's death, I finally nerved myself to read her diaries. I was overwhelmed by the sense of how often and how profoundly she had been unhappy. But I was almost as taken aback when I began to see how, at some point even in the most desolate entry, she will start to think about future plans—not just what she wanted to write, but often books she wanted to read, plays she wanted to see, music she wanted to hear or to listen to again. She begins to make lists of words— "editorial precincts," "headnotes," "scrimshaw," "somatic precondition," "marbled paper"—or of quotations—Gertrude Stein: "poetry is nouns, prose is verbs"—or odd facts—"(?) first depiction of graffiti: Gerard Houckgeest (1600–1661)—'The Tomb of Willem the Silent in the Nieuwe Kerk in Delft': graffiti at the base of column—stick figure w/hat, in red." Before too long, she is outlining a new project, talking herself back into the world she had constructed for herself.

She was aware of all of this, I believe, and knew it to be both her strength and her curse. In a journal entry from the early eighties, my mother declares that "I write the way I live [and] my life is full of quotations." Then she adds: "Change it." But she never did.

How could she have? Her diaries confirm what I always believed about her, which was that no matter what happened to my mother, no matter how defeated or trapped or thwarted or misunderstood she might feel at any given moment, she would eventually right herself, eyes set firmly on the future, on what would come next. It wasn't just ambition, or curiosity, or vanity, or the wish to act on the deepest of her ambitions, set in adolescence, that she sometimes described as "surpassing" herself. On one level, it was all of those things, but I have come to think that deeper still what sustained and nourished my mother was an almost childlike sense of wonder. That was what propelled her from project to project, voyage to voyage, artistic performance to artistic performance. It may sound stupid to put it this way, but my mother simply could never get her fill of the world. And then, in what, despite her age, must have seemed like the midst of all that, it was time to die.

If there really were some benevolent god or world

spirit inclined to meddle in the affairs of human beings, or at least to shelter them from what they most feared, my mother would not have died slowly and painfully from MDS but suddenly from a massive heart attack— the death that all of us who, like my mother (and like me), are crippled by the fear of extinction must yearn for. Sometimes I have actually even visualized it: at one moment there my mother is, talking about something she had just seen, or was about to see, or had just read, or reread, or was about to reread, or some place she planned soon to travel to, and then at the next—or within a few moments, anyway—she would be gone. There would have been no time for her to be frightened, nor to be crushed by the fact that she hadn't done the work she'd most wanted to do, or live the life she'd wanted to live ("Too often," she writes in one of her journals, "I sink to the occasion"). She would not have had the time to mourn herself and to become physically unrecognizable at the end even to herself, let alone humiliated posthumously by being "memorialized" that way in those carnival images of celebrity death taken by Annie Leibovitz.

Of course, my mother did not get swift release in death any more than she got good health in life. Instead, she who feared isolation and had the most terrible difficulties connecting with people had the loneliest of deaths. It is on that account, and that account alone, that I find myself wondering whether the false hope those close to her strived so hard to provide her with in the end consoled her or just increased that isolation. But, though this is one more pavilion in that palace of guilt that I think almost all those who survive sooner or later erect for their dead loved ones, my choice and that of everyone who was close to my mother in those last months—certainly once it was clear that the transplant had not gone well—boiled down to hope or truth. The choice seemed clear at the time, and clearer still now. If that meant making myself an accomplice in an illusion, it was not a steep price to pay for any measure of solace. And there was always that tiny, remote chance that she might survive, if only for a little while longer, that her (unspoken) plea for a little more time, unlike Madame du Barry's on the threshold of the guillotine, would actually be granted.

And yet I know that some of my mother's doctors, particularly at Fred Hutchinson in Seattle, found this troubling. On one level, I can understand. Doctors who specialize in caring for the dying often use the expression "reframing hope," by which they mean helping mortally ill people find a way to shift from hoping to live to connecting in some final, profound way with their loved ones—saying what they had never said, asking what they had never dared ask. I have no idea how much dying people are consoled by this "reframing." I assume some are strengthened by it, though even in such cases I can't help feeling that "hope" is far too strong and sentimental a word. I hear something of the same wishful thinking that overwhelms when I hear the word "closure." There is no "closure" on offer for the death of someone you love. Of that, at least, I'm certain. And I very much doubt that "hope," framed or reframed, offers much to someone trying to organize his or her thoughts and feelings in the shadow of extinction.

The cynic in me wonders if "reframing hope" isn't one of those terms created more for the benefit of the doctors treating the dying than for the dying themselves. Or perhaps my skepticism is one more emblem of the gap between the scientific and the nonscientific worldview. After all, for the doctors at the Hutch extinction is a daily experience, much as they wish it were otherwise and their work is dedicated to transforming the current reality of cancer treatment. One wrote me much later that, in his experience, my mother's "rage against the dying of the light was atypical—given the [actual] state of affairs, all that she had gone through, and the incontrovertible prognosis. The vast majority of individuals in that situation stop fighting and accept the inevitable because of either fatigue, fear, and/or the hope of making the last bit of limited time memorable for those they'll leave behind."

Self-evidently, I am in no position to say what is or is not typical at the end of life. But I hardly think my mother was unique. As I have written this memoir, I have been reading what other writers have said about death and it seems to me that few of them were any more resigned to extinction than my mother was. And for all the ways in which writers are untypical, surely they are not as untypical as all that! Surely, as he lay dying in Memorial Sloan-Kettering in 1987, the great Israeli poet Abba Kovner spoke for more than just poets when he wrote:

> Soon
> soon we shall know
> if we have learned to accept that the stars
> do not go out when we die.

Almost two years after my mother died, I went to see Dr. John Niederhuber, then newly appointed as head of the National Cancer Institute. Most of our conversation revolved around what the NCI was doing, the future of cancer research (above all the question of how and what to fund). But at a certain moment, Niederhuber began to speak of his wife's death from a recurrence of breast cancer. She, too, had been cancer free for a very long time, and then, after twenty years of normal blood counts and scans that showed no recurrence of disease, she fell ill again. Niederhuber spoke of all this quietly, with great simplicity and great emotion. Describing his wife's last day, he said, "There she was, practically a skeleton, and yet what she spoke to me about was getting in better physical shape so that when she underwent the next experimental treatment she would be strong enough to tolerate it."

Denial? Perhaps that would be an end-of-life doctor's term for it. But for me, the word means little and matters less. As the old Oxbridge joke has it, "what's true is obvious, and what isn't obvious isn't true." For my mother, as for John Niederhuber's wife, extinction was unimaginable. She could only think in terms of the next step. This was true to the very end, as Marcel van den Brink, chief of the Adult Bone Marrow Transplant Service at Memorial Sloan-Kettering, later confirmed to me. "In her final weeks," he wrote in an e-mail, "she would often complain of 'the pain all over,' and say 'I don't want any more.' However, if I tried to focus on palliation, she would immediately bring the discussion back from this deep despair to when and how we could continue her therapy."

Thanks to van den Brink and Stephen Nimer, the therapy was continued. "Always assuming [the treatment] is not medically futile," Nimer told me at some point during my mother's last weeks, "if I can carry out my patient's wishes, I want to do that." By then, my mother was largely unable to make her wishes known, though she had moments of clarity ("protective hibernation" was the way one of the Memorial Sloan-Kettering psychiatrists described her state). But neither van den Brink nor Nimer nor I doubted that had she been able to make her wishes known, my mother would have said that she wanted to fight for her life to the very end.

And yet, she had the death that somewhere she must have come to believe that *other* people had from cancer—the death where knowledge meant nothing, the will to fight meant nothing, the skill of the doctors meant nothing. She had the death that she had anticipated having, when, just after she was diagnosed, she had said to me, "This time I don't feel special." Of course, none of us are special. Of course, that poster that had so struck me on the New York City subways of my youth, the one that read "To the other guy, you're the other guy," had been a great deal closer to the reality of human unimportance than my mother's steely resolve. And yet feeling special is part of what makes us human.

Perhaps a good Buddhist can really take in the full reality of human unimportance and still remain compassionate, though if the American Buddhists I knew in my twenties are at all representative, the creed is more often a rationale for existential selfishness than self-abnegation in any real sense of the term. At the very least, such wisdom is very rare. And what my mother strived to do, what any creative writer strives to do (I think this is true of many other vocations as well, but here I restrict myself to what I know—the family olive oil business, as I sometimes thought of it when I was young), is to present themselves, their thoughts, their insights, their knowledge—distill it all and send it out into the world. How to do that and at the same time fully take in the real measure of one's own insignificance? My mother couldn't do it, obviously. But for all the particularities of her character, I have come to doubt that any of us can.

IX

THERE ARE TIMES when I wish I could have died in her place. Survivor's guilt? Doubtless that is part of the story. But only a part. In any case, I do not mean it as melodramatically as it might sound. This is not an out-take from *A Tale of Two Cities,* and I am not Sydney Carton. Nor, overwhelming as they are when such thoughts engulf me, are they by any means the sole or even the principal reaction to my mother's death that I have struggled with since her passing. But I cannot shake the feelings, either, and in many ways they remain the strongest if not the deepest feelings that hold me in their grasp. It is not a question of the fear of death, for I am by no means sure I am any less terrified of or unreconciled to extinction than she was. Nor do they derive from some rare degree of filial devotion. I have preferred to write as little as possible of my relations with my mother in the last decade of her life, but suffice it to say that they were often strained and at times very difficult. But to each according to his needs, as Marx rightly said. Between someone who is in love with the world—and how she loved just . . . being!—and someone who is not, the appropriate outcome, were such a thing on offer, is self-evident. And to say that my mother both enjoyed and made better use of the world than I have ever done or will do is simply a statement of fact.

This question of how unfair to her it is that she is gone and why I'm still here for a bit longer comes into my head at the most improbable moments. While making an inventory of some of her personal things shortly after she died, I found in her wallet a thick wad of cards—memberships to museums, performance spaces, and frequent-flyer programs, and cards from restaurants. That wallet itself was like a set of future itineraries. These days, the thought occurs to me frequently when I am passing one of the many new buildings that have gone up in New York since my mother's death. "How she would have hated *that*," I find myself thinking. Or, "What a pity she never got to see *that*. It would have interested her." At other times, I will read a review of a new Chinese restaurant in the *New York Times* and think how she would have clipped the article and made her way to it. Or I see that a favorite performance group of hers is starting their new season and I think, "I can't believe she isn't here to see them."

But of course, I do believe it. Absolutely. For while I have heard many people insist after the death of a loved one that they can't believe that the person is really gone and sometimes even that they keep fantasizing that the person is not really dead at all but rather that he or she will be coming back at some point, through no particular strength of my own I was never vulnerable to this illusion. Perhaps it was because my mother's dying was so protracted. What seemed to her (and rightly) like such a swift and terrible spiral downward afforded those of us around her almost too much time to prepare ourselves for the finality of her passing. As she died, we swam alongside her, in the sea of her own death, watching her die. Then she did die. And speaking for myself, I find that I am still swimming in that sea.

I REALIZE that I have written about everything except how she died. Strange what one finds most difficult.

The day before she died, she asked, "Is David here?" Her eyes were clenched shut. By then, she was not speaking to any of those around her except to ask to be turned in her bed, or given water, or to ask for the nurse. But she had been speaking a lot, in a low tone, and seemingly to herself, about her mother and about a great love of a much earlier period of her life, Joseph Brodsky.

"Yes, David's right next to your bed," I remember hearing someone say. "Yes, I'm here," I remember hearing myself say.

My mother did not open her eyes, or move her head. For a moment, I thought that she had fallen back to sleep. But after a pause, she said, "I want to tell you . . ."

That was all she said. She gestured vaguely with one emaciated hand and then let it drop onto the coverlet. I think she did fall back to sleep then. These were the last words my mother spoke to me.

If, as I believe, she had imagined herself special, my mother's last illness cruelly exposed the frailty of that conceit. It was merciless in the toll of pain and fear that it exacted. My mother, who feared extinction above all else, was in anguish over its imminence. Shortly before she died, she turned to one of the nurses aides—a superb woman who cared for her like her own daughter—and said, "I'm going to die," and then began to weep. And yet, if her illness was merciless, her death was merciful. About forty-eight hours before the end, she began to fail, complaining of generalized low-grade pain (a sign, it seems, that the leukemia was back in her bloodstream). The doctors found that she had an infection and told me that given the compromised state of her immune system there was little chance that her body could stave off the infection. She remained intermittently lucid for about another day, though her throat was so abraded that she could barely speak audibly and she was confused. I *feel* she knew I was there, but I am not at all sure. She said she was dying; she asked if she was crazy.

By Monday afternoon, she had left us, though she was still alive. Preterminal, the doctors call it. It was not that she wasn't there or was wholly unconscious; she was neither. But she had gone to a place deep within herself, to some last redoubt of her being, at least as I imagine it. What she took in I will never know, but she could no longer make much contact, if, indeed, she even wanted to. I and the others who were at her side left around 11:00 p.m. and went home to get a few hours' sleep. At 3:30 a.m., a nurse called. My mother was failing. In the room, we found her hooked up to an oxygen machine. Her blood pressure had already dropped into a perilous zone and was dropping steadily, her pulse was weakening, and the oxygen in her blood was growing thinner.

For an hour and a half, my mother seemed to hold her own. Then, she began the last step. I had called Stephen Nimer at 6:00 a.m. and he came over immediately. He stayed with her throughout her death.

And her death was easy, as deaths go, I mean, and in the sense that she was in little pain and little visible anguish. She simply went. First, she took a deep breath; there was a pause of forty seconds, such an agonizing, open-ended time if you are watching a human being end; then another deep breath. This went on for no more than a few minutes. Then the pause became permanence, the person ceased to be, and Stephen Nimer said, "She's gone."

A few days after my mother died, Stephen Nimer sent me an e-mail. "I think about Susan all the time," he wrote. And then he added, "We have to do better."

I SHALL BE forever grateful for that e-mail. And yet, if I am being completely honest, I am not entirely sure I know how to think about it anymore. As I understand him, Stephen Nimer was expressing both his compassion and his hope as a scientist and a physician that one day he and his colleagues would have better treatments for the blood cancer patients like my mother to whom they devoted their lives and whose chances of survival, in so many cases, are still so slight. And I honor him and will always love him for that. But because his words (rightly) address what we die of and not, of course, the fact that we die, there is a sense in which they don't really touch on my mother's deep refusal of death itself—a refusal in which, despite what some of her doctors in Seattle supposed, she was anything but alone. Yes, of course we have to do better, and I don't doubt that great doctors like Stephen Nimer will do better. But with the greatest respect, the brute fact of mortality means that there are limits on how much better we can realistically expect to do.

I am not even remotely smart enough to resolve any of this, even in my own mind. But some facts seem inescapable. Fantasies of immortality notwithstanding, most biologists agree that the human life span is more or less finite. And if so many people die of cancer today, doctors say that this is at least in part because we are not dying of other diseases when we are younger. Presumably, this means that if oncologists really do become more successful at treating cancer and, to use the triumphalist phrase one encounters in the literature handed out in many cancer centers, manage to turn at least many cancers into "chronic" illnesses rather than mortal ones, what people will then have to die of will be something else—something about which we will not do better, something that cannot be long remitted.

In the end, that is the question that haunts me. Had Stephen Nimer been able to save my mother's life, would she have been reconciled to dying of something else later on? Are any of us, when it's our turn? In her bleak, extraordinary end-of-life journal, Marguerite Duras states flatly, "I cannot reconcile myself to being nothing." It is a sentence that my mother could have written as well, she who so loved just being alive. In one of her journal entries, she takes all this on frontally. "Death is unbearable unless you can get beyond the 'I,'" she writes. But she who could do so many things in her life could never do that.

Clearly, some people have this gift, or, more properly, can find their way to it. As he lay dying in his room in the Charité Hospital in Berlin, Bertolt Brecht wrote an extraordinary series of final poems. In the last of them, he looked out his window at a bird in a nearby tree whose call he found beautiful. Brecht writes of thinking that after he is dead, the bird will be alive, in its tree, warbling its beautiful call. The wisdom of the poem lies in the artist reconciling himself to that fact, reveling in the beauty of the world, resigning himself to his own transience, his own evanescence. "For nothing can be wrong with me," he writes, "if I myself am nothing. Now I managed to enjoy the song of every blackbird after me too."

But viscerally, I do not believe that my mother could love a world without herself, much as the moralist in her would have despised herself for not doing so. Because she could not free herself from her hope about life, about the world—despite her intermittent melancholia, I always thought that she was first and foremost the very incarnation of hope—she never really had a chance of freeing herself from her terrible fear of extinction, of not being. Where I do not know if I behaved well or badly, and, far more importantly, helpfully, by trying to buttress that hope throughout the course of her illness, I was fully conscious at the time that the more she hoped, the harder it would be for my mother to die. But to talk with her as if it were more likely that she was going to die than to live seemed certain to increase her fear and pain. It was a decision that I rationalized with the argument that it was too late for her to abandon hoping, if that was even possible given her nature, and that for her the end of hope would not mean the end of fear—Brecht's epiphany in his "Charité" poem—but just more despair and panic and meaninglessness. Surely it was better to die hoping than cowering in terror, as I feared she might have done. But I am anything but certain that I did the right thing, and, in my bleaker moments, wonder if in fact I might not have made things worse for her by endlessly refilling that poisoned chalice of hope.

To say that I would have wished for her Brecht's calm at his end, rather than Duras' panic, is at best an expression of love and probably is little better than a hollow sentiment. Certainly, sentiments like these did nothing to help her, and she was rightly contemptuous of them, seeing them for what they were: a consolation for those who will go on living. Of course, the skeptic in me wonders what it was really like for Brecht or those who loved him in those last days. If his poem is to be believed, he had an easier death than my mother did. But then, that is the solace of art, and also its mendacity. Art had always been my mother's solace, too. But not the least of the cruelties of her death was that what had sustained, inspired, and informed her in life made it so much harder for her to die.

I still cannot believe there was nothing I could do to help.

EPILOGUE

My mother lies buried in the Montparnasse Cemetery in Paris. If you enter it through the main gate on the Boulevard Edgar Quinet, you will find Simone de Beauvoir's grave almost directly on your right as you head toward my mother's burial plot. Whatever remains of Samuel Beckett lies under a plain gray granite slab a hundred meters from the black polished slab that covers the bones and whatever else now remains of the embalmed corpse that was once an American writer named Susan Sontag, 1933–2004. My mother's friend the writer Emile Cioran's grave is two hundred meters or so in the opposite direction. Sartre, Raymond Aron, and, most famously, Baudelaire, are buried there, too.

The graves are easy to find as there are maps at the cemetery entrance directing visitors to the gravesites of the celebrated. In short, Montparnasse is the most literary of cemeteries, a veritable Parnassus. Except, of course, that it's nothing of the sort—not unless you believe in spirits or the Christian fairy tale of resurrection, anyway—and for a simple reason: the men and women in question no longer exist The best one can do, and I'm not sure I believe a word of it, is say along with Bei Dao that "as long as one's thoughts are spoken and written down, they'll form another life, they won't perish with the flesh."

Does this constitute remembrance? Simone de Beauvoir certainly did not think so when she wrote in her memoir of her own mother's death that "whether you think of it as heavenly or as earthly, if you cling to living immortality is no consolation for death."

My mother was equally unpersuaded and unconsoled. And yet she was herself an inveterate visitor of graveyards—Mt. Auburn in Boston, Colón in Havana, La Recoleta in Buenos Aires, Highgate in London, and, of course, Montparnasse, to name only the most celebrated. Given her chill, clammy fear of extinction, I never entirely understood this. For while she was interested in memento mori, and for decades kept a human skull on a shelf behind her desk alongside art nouveau knickknacks and photographs of her private pantheon of writers she admired most, I don't believe by visiting these cemeteries she meant to rub her own nose in her mortality. Instead, like the many literary tourists one sees in Montparnasse Cemetery today—the ones who leave Metro tickets on Beckett's grave and lately, I have found, the small polished stones she loved and collected as well as flowers on my mother's—she was paying homage and, in doing so, keeping alive that second life of art.

In reality, though, my decision to bury my mother in Montparnasse had little to do either with literature or even with her lifelong love of Paris, rapturous as it was. The decision was mine alone—that much her will had stipulated—and I had to bury her somewhere—she had a horror of cremation. But since she believed to the end that she was going to survive her cancer, and therefore had seen no reason to leave any specific instructions or even to express any wishes on the matter, I had no idea what those wishes might have been. We had no ceremonies of good-bye, to use Beauvoir's great phrase. And without her voice to guide me, I had nothing to go on. It was as if she had died suddenly, in a car accident or a plane crash, rather than slowly, incrementally, horribly of MDS.

THE ONLY concrete thing she ever asked for was that a late Beethoven quartet she had loved since adolescence be played at her memorial. But that was an idea that dated back to her adolescence, and as such seemed almost unconnected to her real death. So I improvised, all the while wondering, as I still wonder, if I was doing the right thing.

The cemeteries of New York are ugly, and the particular one where her own father is buried is one of the ugliest of all of them. Besides, my mother had not known of it until very late in her life and, as far as I know, only visited it once, even if her father figured repeatedly in the inwardly directed talk of her final days—talk that seemed to carom freely between lament, settling of accounts, and personal history. And I knew that my mother felt no particular connection to the other American cities—Tucson, Los Angeles, Chicago, and Boston—in which she had lived. That left Paris, for so long her second home. Or so I reasoned, to the extent that I was capable of reason in the immediate aftermath of my mother's death. In any case, Paris was also a second home to many of my mother's friends, and as far as I can see, graves are for the living if they are for anything at all.

And so I had my mother's body shipped from Kennedy Airport in New York to Paris aboard the same Air France evening flight she had taken literally hundreds of times during her life. It was our last trip together. I remember thinking, "I am taking my mother to Paris for the last time." The journey began over the Atlantic, me in my window seat, the tranquilizers having zero effect, she in the hold. And it ended in the Volvo hearse that moved smoothly from the funeral home at the edge of the city to Montparnasse, along the boulevards she had known so well and loved so ardently. The Périphérique to the Opéra, the Opéra to the Madeleine, the Madeleine to the Place de la Concorde; across the Seine into Saint-Germain—"her" neighborhood from the time she first set foot in Paris in 1957, aged twenty-four—and past the National Assembly, the Boulevard Raspail to the Boulevard Montparnasse, and finally along the Boulevard Edgar Quinet to the cemetery gates. I took my mother on one last, sweeping ride through Paris, and then I buried her.

And so it ended. As her corpse was lowered into the grave, and I knelt at the edge of the burial hole, I felt she was still there. Today, when I go to visit my mother's grave, I do not know what to do besides tidy up a bit (me tidying up for my mother!—a preposterous reversal of roles). In any case, the cemetery gardeners do an excellent job, as do the many visitors to the gravesite. But I do not believe she is there, or anywhere else of course, and so I rarely stay long. I arrive, walking quickly past Beauvoir, past Beckett. And once I've arrived I stare for a few moments. Then I kneel, kiss the granite slab, and get back up on my feet. And then I go—hurriedly, confusedly—past Beckett and Beauvoir again if I retrace my steps, and past Cioran if I do not. It is not just that I have nothing intelligent to say: I am incapable of thought.

And not only at graveside. Looking back on my mother's death, I have few thoughts and many regrets. Mostly, I feel guilty—the default position of the survivor. I wish that I had complied more with her wishes during her lifetime, more or less in all regards. I wish I could have suppressed my own interests in the furtherance of hers. Which is only to say that I wish that I had lived, while she was alive and well, with the image of her death at the forefront of my consciousness. Of course, I know full well that these are idle wishes—wishes that only someone truly without ego could imagine themselves in a position to fulfill. Their childishness, their bogus saintliness, their masochism, appalls me, and yet I am unable (or is it unwilling?) to let them go entirely. No matter how much you care about someone, you cannot act as if you are always attending them at their deathbed. It is back to that remark of Kierkegaard's that Jerome Groopman is so fond of quoting: life must be lived prospectively but can only be understood retrospectively. The problem is that, by then, it is usually too late.

What does that leave? Closure? Again, I do not believe for an instant that there is any such thing. If there is any . . . easing, it is probably that as time passes, all the grief, all the layers of one's feelings eventually "migrate" somewhere. Or perhaps we become accustomed to our grief and, as it becomes increasingly familiar, increasingly part of the emotional landscape, it becomes a dullness. But there is no closure; no forgetting is on offer. One mourns those one has loved who have died until one joins them. It happens soon enough.

In the meantime, what to do? In *The Gay Science*, Nietzsche describes "the melancholy happiness" he derives from the spectacle of human beings loving life and rejecting the thought of death. It is as if he loves them for their gallantry since they will all be extinguished sooner rather than later. His observation consoles me in some way I can neither entirely explain nor entirely justify. In one of her own journals, in an entry written during the period when she was receiving chemotherapy at Memorial Sloan-Kettering for her breast cancer, my mother enjoined herself to "be cheerful, be stoic, be tranquil." And then she added, "In the valley of sorrow, spread your wings."

This was not the death she died. But in the end, I think that what she said—whether she entirely believed it or not; whether any of us can come to entirely believe it or not—is the best that can be said of old mortality.

In the valley of sorrow, spread your wings.

ABOUT THE AUTHOR

DAVID RIEFF is a contributing writer to the *New York Times Magazine*. He is the author of seven previous books, including the acclaimed *At the Point of a Gun: Democratic Dreams and Armed Intervention; A Bed for the Night: Humanitarianism in Crisis;* and *Slaughterhouse: Bosnia and the Failure of the West.* He lives in New York City.